The
EYES
Have It

The EYES Have It

A Self-help Manual for Better Vision

Earlyne Chaney

Samuel Weiser, Inc.
York Beach, Maine

First published in 1987 by
Samuel Weiser, Inc.
Box 612
York Beach, Maine 03910

Library of Congress Cataloging in Publication Data

Chaney, Earlyne.
    The eyes have it.

    1. Vision.   2. Orthoptics.   3. Holistic medicine.
I. Title.
RE51.C445   1987   617.7   86-23438
ISBN 0-941683-03-6

Cover illustration © K. Kruidenier, 1979

Typeset in 11 point Palatino
Printed in the United States of America

CONTENTS

INTRODUCTION

Poets remind us that the eyes are the windows of the soul. We have come to realize there is more than just imagination in that metaphor. They are also the mirrors of health. Nature has created an organ, a vessel, a channel keyed and adjusted to a precision unmatched by man's ultimate machinery. The most complex camera, television mechanism, telescope, or microscope is put to shame by the peerless precision of the human eye. Sight is the incomparable—the only—human sense that can reach beyond the Earth to bring us knowledge of other worlds. So open your eyes to a new awareness. See—not only with your eyes but with your soul. Many worlds await your beholding.

The material here comes from years of training and many sources to which I am indebted:

• the famous Bates system of training the eyes to see. Bates was a medical doctor turned healer.

• the writings and practices of a dear chiropractor-naturopath who brought about more natural cures than any medical doctor I ever heard of. I called him Dr. Som. Many of the home, herbal, and natural folk remedies were taught to me by Dr. Som.

• my years of yogic training, encompassing many of the disciplines given me by my "unseen" teachers from Higher Worlds.

• hours of research into the latest offerings of medical science toward helping us "see" better through medical aids and "breakthroughs."

You seekers of better sight must choose for yourselves the best method for your own personal benefit. As for me, I select techniques from all systems from time to time—and happily use whatever and whichever appeals at the moment.

I believe the methods of palming and sunning and the drills presented by Dr. Bates to be unsurpassed. So I use them intermittently. But during my early morning yoga session I faithfully practice yogic techniques. Both systems have served me well.

I deplore using glasses as a crutch. But I do not join the vociferous writers who lambaste all people who wear glasses. I wholeheartedly endorse every effort to improve eyesight; but I certainly don't look askance at those who wear glasses, nor do I consider them too indolent to try for correction.

The market is overrun with books about "perfect vision without glasses." Not this one. This one suggests *the way to healthy eyes*. I don't deplore wearing glasses—in fact I give thanks there are such things. What I deplore is the way people automatically submit to eye problems without making every effort to heal them or to keep their eyes healthy. I deplore brainwashing that makes millions believe glasses are the norm—"for one my age." I deplore the way youngsters are put behind glasses rather than on a corrective program. I deplore that the optical profession refuses to recognize that there exists a means of aiding problem eyes other than wearing glasses. I truly believe that every patient should be given advice on improvement and that the doctor should be ready to fit that patient in weaker and weaker glasses until the patient, following the doctor's program, can discard glasses entirely.

True, I have witnessed miracles from following a good purification program, through which many discard their glasses. But certainly not the majority. So, I'd like to make it clear right at the outset that this is not another of those "follow my procedure and throw away your glasses" books. This book will guide you toward *the art of seeing*—with or without glasses. It points toward health for the eyes, with or without glasses. It offers preventive measures. It offers all sorts of aids and advice.

Do I wear glasses? Well, yes and no. I have a pair of glasses and a pair of contact lenses. Most of the time, I forget to wear either of them—and I see just fine. Then suddenly there comes a cycle when my eyesight needs a boost, and I find myself seeking my glasses.

I usually wear my contacts when I lecture, even though I may not really need them. Why? Because I want to see the faces of my audience really well, even those far in the back. I like a good straight eye contact. I use "eye rays" as healing rays all during my seminars, especially during my healing services, so I sometimes wear the contacts to better align with the eye rays of my audience.

I wear them also because someone is always thrusting reading matter into my hands with a request that I hurriedly read something. I can't be constantly reaching for glasses just in case the print may be fine. I wear my contacts with deep gratitude that God gave us the wisdom and the know-how to produce them.

I *still* practice eye exercises. I *still* watch my vegetarian diet. I *still* think love thoughts. I *still* try for never-never glasses and achieve it a great share of the time.

But the main point of this book is *health for the eyes*. If, in achieving this health, you can discard your glasses, wonderful! That's a double blessing. Do try!

Part 1

THE ART OF SEEING

Health is that state of mind in which the body is not consciously present to us; the state in which it is a joy to think, to feel, to be, to see.

— Sir Andrew Clark, M.D
Physician to Queen Victoria

THE WINDOWS OF THE WHOLE PERSON

Note that the title of this book is *The Eyes Have It*. It is meant as an aid to sharpen your awareness as well as your eyes. So before we tackle techniques, I must ask you a question. "See" if you can answer it.

Do you realize you "see" with your consciousness and not your eyes?

A cow staked out to graze does not see the beauty of a landscape. Her awareness is only on the grass to eat. You, viewing the same landscape, see with your consciousness. Both the cow and you have eyes—but the conscious awareness in you sees with much more.

Another question: Could it be that by living to the highest potential of our awareness, the highest thought-voltage of our love force, we could "see" without glasses? That we could "see" with our fingertips? That we could "see" the unseen all about us?

It's just a thought. A thought-provoking thought. We'll consider it later. We'll consider first the physiology of the eye and exercises and methods to help you have healthy eyes. Then we'll consider consciousness again—consciousness in a world without glasses.

Stand at a large picture window and view the landscape in daylight. Notice how well you can see without your glasses. See the outline of hills, or any skyline. Don't worry about whether the scene is clear or blurred. Don't worry! Now cease to concentrate on seeing the scene. Think instead of a happy day in the past, or of a very funny story or joke. Suddenly any blur in the outside scene becomes sharp. Your entire vision temporarily becomes sharp and clear. As soon as you direct energy away from the eyes and cease to worry about them, the eyes immediately function properly, especially when thoughts are happy.

The expression of the eyes changes according to the emotions felt in the innermost part of your being. Sympathy, love, compassion, anger, hate, fear—all of these emotions are reflected in the eyes as the state of inner consciousness looks through. This is true of the relaxed normal eye. A more modern aphorism might warn us that, although the eyes *are* windows reflecting the awareness of the soul, there are many types of windows. Because they also reflect the status of human health, eyes are often poor revealers of the soul.

One can never teach health for the eyes only; it must constantly be remembered that the eyes are part of, and involved in, the enitre physical being, the whole person. When health problems manifest anywhere in the body, the eyes are always affected, and usually first. The eyes, then, can be called the windows of the human trinity—the soul, the personality, and the physical body. Pain or discomfort can quickly cause the eye to become a distorted mirror of the soul.

SEEING AND PERCEPTION

"She made me so mad I couldn't see straight!" Don't let anyone continually make you angry, or soon the eyes won't "see straight." Stress! For good vision there must be integration of vision with the evolution of your level of consciousness and awareness. Seeing straight might mean better understanding, cooler coping.

Seeing and perception could be partners; perception is the way we see the world; the way we see our husband or wife; the way we see a dominating parent; the way we see our future; the way we see God. Expanded consciousness—a greater awareness of life's mysteries—could mean better eyesight. A deliverance from the fear of death could "open one's eyes" to both physical and soul vision.

When you *understand* a certain teaching, you say, "I see" or "I see what you mean." You are actually saying, "I perceive your thought. I understand what you are saying." There are myriad ways of seeing.

And then there are those who can "see" with their fingertips, such as Rosa Kuleshova of Russia. She not only "sees" colors and chooses them correctly in blind tests, but she can also read blindfolded. Another, Lena Bleznova, can distinguish colors with her feet. A third, Nadia Lobanova, who is blind, can tell colors at a distance without touching them. With her hands eight inches from the text, she reads large letters, in both the light and the dark.

Others, in America and elsewhere, can select the correct colors in similar circumstances. Such an ability is called *extra-ocular* vision. Perhaps we have a crystalline lens and retina in our sensitive fingertips but don't know it. Perhaps as we unfold our other higher perceptions, we'll find we can see perfectly well with our fingertips even when our eyes can't.

But how does this "second sight" work? Sight has two organs: the eyes and the skin. The skin consists of visual microscopic ocelli distributed over the whole epidermis but especially in the fingertips. The ocelli possess a refracting body, an ocillary retina, an optical fiber.

This second-sight organ must have been originally designed for use in darkness (given that the eyes see only in light). The phenomenon of seeing in darkness is called *nictopia*. The problem is that of focusing peripheral or field vision into homocentric visibility—in other words, closing out all excessive areas to beam in on one small area. The difficulty, then, is not that of extending but of reducing the field of vision. "Paroptic" vision gains in integrity what it must lose of its integrality.

The paroptic vision—that of seeing with the finger-tips—could be a bridge between physical and psychic vision. The diffused peripheral skin vision could be extended as a sky vision, like a telescope focusing on one small space. It could finally project itself beyond space and become psychic clairvoyance.

Receptive and reflective, the paroptic function could explain the so-called "aura" phenomenon. Its absorption of light may awaken in the brain some sensitive organ—a sixth sense organ—that could change the peripheral absorption of light into psychic clairvoyance. Psychic clairvoyance is only an occasional occurrence in the untrained human mind. It could become a permanent psychic faculty through fully developed and trained paroptic vision. Its development could thus follow naturally from that of peripheral illumination.

It is groups of ocelli that form in the primitive eyes of insects, enabling them to see in the dark. This is also true of the cat, which sees perfectly well in the dark.

The theory of research mystics—my theory, at least—is that the human eye has evolved from skin tissue, and therefore the skin cells still retain the latent ability to receive visual impressions. I believe there is a direct connection between the eyes and certain sensitive centers, especially the fingertips and palms. The microscopic nerve organs of the skin are potential eyes.

According to scientists, each cell in our body is a miniature battery with a potential charge of about 1.17 volts. The flow of current in all of the body cells amounts to about 76 amperes. One stroke of a comb through the hair will produce an electrical value of from 8,000 to 10,000 volts.

Feelings of pleasure on any skin area will create an increase in bioelectrical charge in the skin. Feelings of displeasure—negative feelings such as fear, anxiety, irritation—create a decrease in bioelectrical charge. So to establish a positive possibility of seeing, not only with the fingertips but even with better eyesight, one should live in an atmosphere of the highest possible spiritual voltage, an aura of total love and bliss. Much of attaining healthier eyes has to do with recognizing stress and tension in our lives and learning how to relax.

Tension

Worry and fear create inner tension. All negative emotions affect the eyes almost immediately. We are all familiar with such descriptive phrases as "blind with rage," "I saw red I was so mad," "I was so furious I couldn't see straight."

How literally true they are. Rage can tentatively blind one. Anger can redden the eyes, swelling minute minor blood vessels. Anger can cause the vision to blur and "warp," and you actually can't see straight.

Defective eyesight is common among people who are unhappy with their jobs—especially when they feel trapped and unable to change. Bad posture and poor lighting are among the more common physical causes.

Tension is the first enemy of both inner or outer beauty. Stress is always reflected first in the eyes. A soul can easily be misjudged. People can be accused of having "shifty eyes," meaning their dealings with others may be devious. It may be because their eyes hurt from inner tension. They shift their eyes as they would shift a hurting foot, not knowing where to put it. Others, supersensitive to light, may draw their brows down and together, appearing to scowl when they are only uncomfortable. Others may appear cold, unfeeling, even haughty, because their eyes are fixed and staring due to stiff muscles.

Eyes full of tension become a poor mirror for the inner feelings because, through tension, the great inner light is overcast and the eyes become simply physical organs filled with discomfort. We should never be quick to judge people via the eyes. Only when the eye and the overall health are normal can the old adage "as within so without" truly be proved. The soul truly *can* use the normal eye as a mirror.

Tension is always intensified in the eyes, manifesting as tight lids and tight muscles. Tense muscles often create a furrow between the eyebrows in an effort to relieve inner discomfort. Tensed eye muscles then create congestion, which means the circulation of blood and life force is being partially blocked. If the tension continues, the drawn eye muscles cause the eye to appear smaller in its setting. Over a period of time, the lack of life force will even fade the color. Nothing fades the color of the eye more rapidly.

Have you ever noticed how your eyes shine when you are happy? The eyes of a little child sparkle when an unexpected treat or a gift is given. This should be the natural state of your eyes, quick and ready to register your emotions.

Go for a walk or take a bus ride just to observe the eyes of those you meet. Some reflect the sure, unfaltering light of faith, love, hope, and confidence. Most reflect the message of quiet resignation, the sign that the quest has been abandoned, the dreams of earlier years have died. Others reflect hopeless despair. Lack of love will undernourish a soul just as lack of proper food undernourishes the eye. The pain and panic of daily living are reflected in far more eyes than is happiness. Some are fixed and staring as if their owner were far away in thought.

Occasionally one *does* see a vibrant being with sparkling eyes. If questioned, the person is invariably found to be "in love" or "in a state of love." Love is light, and the inner light of love force reflects in the eyes as a sparkle. We'll have more to say concerning light and the eyes in Part 4.

From day to day the degree of tension varies in the eyes, as in the rest of the body. *No eye is normal all the time.* The "normalcy" fluctuates with passing events, but it is most important not to allow stress and tension to attain a state of permanency.

Let's consider some of the tensions that, over a period of time, build up in the eye. They are as varied as the individuals who bear them. First, as we've already stated, is mental strain. Usually, as you mature and assume the responsibilities of life, so your tensions grow. Fears of various levels and aspects become an innate part of the personality—the "normal" fears of life: the fear of failure, fear of what life and its experiences may bring. We face the uncertainty of the future and anxiety for the present. We flash ahead to potential challenges—childbirth, for instance —and wonder about our fortitude. This innate fear of failure is the first great builder of tension—first in the mind, then reflected in the eyes, until the whole face mirrors this inner state. No normal mortal truly ever escapes this inborn fear of personal responsibility, for even the soul itself often questions whether or not it will or can fulfill the mission for which it came.

Sudden shock may temporarily affect vision. The same type of shock that causes the face to blanch and the body to tremble could cause muscle spasm in the eye. Such a spasm may also occur in a highly nervous person after driving in extremely heavy traffic.

There are legions of lesser tensions, more or less temporary in their effect."Look at the clock! Hurry! I'll be late!" "Did I lock the door as I left?" "Have I missed my bus?" "Did I disconnect the iron?" "I'm almost out of gas!" And on and on and on. You may have acquired the faith and knowledge to handle the first group—the hidden inner tensions, the fears of personal responsibility—but we all have these lesser tensions descend upon us daily!

Whether caused by hidden inner tensions of life's fears or by daily stress, tension in the eyes dulls the vision and is often the beginning of organic as well as functional problems. Cataract, glaucoma, and other diseases of the eye are usually caused by tension. If tension can be eliminated, the disease can usually be avoided. We'll talk about several methods of prevention later. One major approach to tension prevention is *relaxation*.

Relaxation

Now that we have considered the negative-tension causes of the eye and whole-person problems, let's investigate a positive and happier view, the one you should emphasize. It is the hopeful thought, the bright outlook, the "light" out-look we are seeking.

No two pairs of eyes are identical; no two have the same degree of either faulty or good vision. Whatever your diffi-culty, *relaxation cannot harm you.*

The art and habit of relaxation are absolutely essential to natural vision. The reason so many people wear glasses is that they have forgotten how to relax. The world is too much with us. The tensions are so constant, our eyes react and suffer the effects of our "quiet panic" about existing in a world seemingly gone mad.

The easiest possible method of being sure tension doesn't build too high in the eye is to close your eyes for brief periods many times a day—short but frequent mo-ments. Cultivate the habit of closing your eyes when read-ing, watching television, sewing, typing, or doing anything else that requires steady viewing. Take a few moments to practice some of the simple exercises in this book—such as "palming"—described in Part 2. Always think happy. Think love. Think tenderness.

Relaxation falls into two categories, passive and dy-namic. *Passive relaxation* is the type you use when, tired, you sit in a chair and completely let go, when you fall across the bed and allow it to hold you instead of your holding it. You are using *dynamic relaxation* if the relaxed feeling of mind and body continues while you go about your active work or play. Active or dynamic relaxation is the type busy people use. After sitting for long hours at work, go for a walk or a swim. It's the kind of relaxation that keeps athletes loose during a game.

The Bates Method of eye correction uses both types of relaxation. First, we seek to put the body in a state of com-fort and ease. The active working mind is quieted down by *the palming drill*—which blocks out light by using the palms. Often it is remarked after palming, "I almost went to sleep."

At times of extreme nervousness it is best to introduce active relaxing drills before palming. They bring into play some of the large body muscles, almost tiring them. The muscular activity tends to quiet the nerves, making it easier to sit quietly and palm the eyes for whatever length of time is necessary for best results. This method is also used successfully with active children. *It is the ability to employ these two forms of relaxation interchangeably that enables the eye to be restored to its proper functioning: not with exercise but with the proper use of relaxation.*

In summing up these remarks on tension and relaxation, we arrive at this conclusion: Relaxation and normalcy of eye, mind, and body are closely related. Not only do various functional disturbances of the eye spring from continued tensions, but tension has been most often at the root of organic trouble as well.

It is not only in the eye that tension does its deadly work but throughout the whole mind and body. Witness the rapid growth in popularity of tranquilizers. Psychiatrists and counselors are in demand because of nervous tensions in both young and old. Many have established a cycle: nerve tension, which brings frustration, which produces additional nerve tension. Many diseases of the body are not only caused by tension but are nurtured by it. Practice of these mechanical aids for relaxation, while applying some of the principles leading toward quietness of mind and soul, helps you sleep without tranquilizers and do your work without the so-called happiness pills. Nor will you need to take your problems—many, if not most, induced by tensions—to a counselor.

PHYSIOLOGY OF THE EYE

Before we discuss common eye ailments, and the subsequent exercises for better eye health contained in this book, it's necessary for you to familiarize yourself with the basic structure of your eyes so you can understand how they work. There are three aspects of the eye that we will focus on:

• the *fovea centralis*, which is the sharpest center of sight in the eye;

• the muscular structure of the eye, so we can better understand the causes of nearsightedness, farsightedness, and astigmatism;

• the crystalline lens, which focuses our vision.

The Fovea Centralis

Many question whether or not eye exercises can benefit the eyes, especially the drills taught by Dr. Bates. What must be understood is that the drills are not for the purpose of exercising the eyes. The principal purpose is to restore movement deep within the eye. Figure 1 shows a diagram of an eye so you can see the areas that we will discuss. The only part of the eye that sees with perfect perception is at the *center* of the retinal nerve tissue. It is a small yellow spot called the *macula lutea*. This center point is as minute as the head of a pin. In the very center of this spot is a small depression called the *fovea centralis*, the point that, when properly focused, gives the sharpest picture to the eye. This is the true center of sight.

When you focus on a small area of an object, you are using the fovea point. The eye could be likened to a bowl whose sides slant upward, or an arena with a small field. The fovea, the dot of perfect vision, is at the bottom of the field-arena. This is the only part of the eye that has strong clear vision. It sees a central object, like a rose in a vase, while the surrounding objects are seen secondarily.

All parts of the retina have seeing ability, but the vision is not as sharp as at the fovea. The dimmer vision is called the *peripheral* vision, the field vision. Example: You are looking at the rose in the vase and focusing your attention and the point of sight on it. At the same time you see the chairs and other objects around the flower.

This little fovea centralis has a natural movement of seventy times a second and, unknown to you, moves as a tiny paint brush over the object on which you are focusing. You are unconsciously using your eyes as paintbrushes, not as blotters. You are not trying to see all things equally well. That would produce a stare. And staring is harmful.

We shall constantly refer to the macula lutea and the fovea throughout the book.

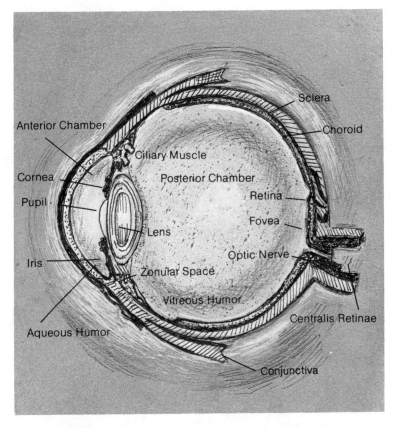

Figure 1. The normal eye. Note the location of the retina, the lens, the optic nerve and the fovea.

Muscle Structure

To understand both the voluntary and involuntary functions of the eye, it is necessary to know something of its
muscle structure. First of all, it is well to remember:

- Myopia, or nearsightedness, is difficulty in seeing
things at a distance.

- Presbyopia, or farsightedness, is difficulty in seeing
things close at hand, such as when reading.

- Astigmatism, deemed incurable, is caused by a curvature in the front part of the eye, the cornea, which is more
acutely curved than the eyeball.

There are six muscles through which the eye functions.
Figure 2 shows the location of the muscles. Four of the
muscles extend from the front of the eye to the back of the
eye, from near the cornea in front to the bony structure at
the back of the eyeball. They are distributed over the eye,
one above, one below, and one on each side. They are called
recti muscles.

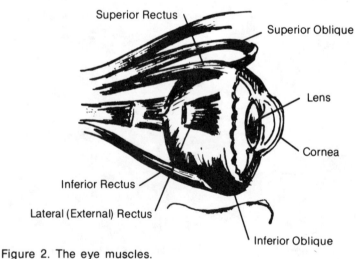

Figure 2. The eye muscles.

The other two muscles circle the eye obliquely, thus acquiring the name *oblique muscles*. One of these oblique muscles is attached to the sclera at the lower side of the eyeball, the other to the upper side of the eyeball. One portion of these muscles is voluntary and is the part used to turn the eye up and down and in and out. It is possible to strain these muscles with unwise, sharp movement such as unaccustomed exercise, just as it is possible to strain or sprain an arm or ankle. A sprained eye muscle will probably produce no permanent damage, but it is inconvenient and most painful, as is any other sprained muscle.

At the place where the muscles are attached to the eye, action is involuntary. The voluntary and involuntary actions are performed by the same muscles. Dr. Bates proved in his work that the accommodation (focusing for near and far seeing) is not dependent on the lens of the eye, for eyes with the lens removed due to a cataract operation were taught to accommodate by the action of the involuntary muscles. The eye is like a camera, the entire eye lengthening in axis for close reading by aid of the oblique muscles, or flattening or shortening by aid of the recti muscles. Dr. Bates found tension in this involuntary action to be the cause of impaired vision for both nearsightedness (myopia) or farsightedness (presbyopia).

When tension or strain in the mind or body is picked up by the eye, these voluntary muscles are stiff and rigid. They are unable to flatten the eyeball for distance or elongate it for near viewing. The tension may be worse one way or the other. It is possible to have poor distant vision and good vision at the near point. The failure to see at the close point, such as when reading, is often associated with advancing years. Nearsightedness seems more prevalent with younger people. However, some persons may have both.

The six muscles around the eyes could be likened to rubber bands. They have been so attached to the front and back of the eye that one pair of muscles pulling forward from the back opposes the backward pull from the front.

The eyeball could be likened to a pliable object caught in a sling drawn taut. The eye can rotate in all directions according to the slack and tension of the two "rubber band" muscles holding it in traction. There are several such slings composed of "rubber band" muscles, the traction of which holds the eye balanced.

When far vision is desired, the pliable eyeball becomes flattened in front, producing longsightedness under normal opposing tensions. When this tension is reduced, the eye lengthens and shortsightedness results, permitting near vision. This is called accommodation—the ability to change focus rapidly. Certain muscles cannot turn the eye in one direction unless opposing muscles relax their tension, much as a rubber band would relax its tautness. Certain muscles, called converging muscles, cannot turn the eye inward or outward unless opposing muscles relax their natural tension.

It is impossible to relax one part of the eye and not another. Outer muscles as well as the interior of the eye benefit from relaxation. When an eye is taught to "look easy," as we shall show in the drills, when it is unafraid of light and rested by palming, then the little fovea at the center of sight is released to do its seventy-times-per-second painting. The involuntary muscles perform with normal ease. Even those tiny muscles around the eyes and those controlling the lids are loosened and freed from their tension. Since the eyes are part of the entire body, impaired vision is usually due to some defective mental or organic function within.

Eyes do not actually see. They are perfect color television aerials. As aerials, they are incredible receivers of myriad wavelengths of light. These wavelengths are transmitted by the eye-aerials to two "television screens" in the brain, located in the back of the head. They are called the visual centers of the brain (see figure 3).

For every one of your five senses—seeing, hearing, feeling, tasting, smelling—there is a brain center, a collec-

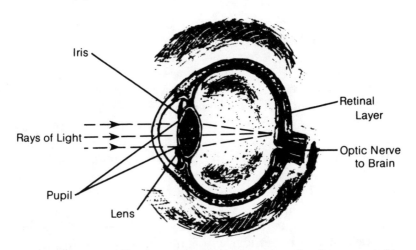

Figure 3. The eye, like the camera that it is, sees only when exposed to light. When light rays strike the eyes, a chemical change occurs in the retina that stimulates impulses that travel through the optic nerve to the brain center near the back of the head. Only then can you "see" with your eyes.

tion of brain cells related to that particular sense. The two related to seeing are the two visual centers at the back of the head. An object is first registered on the retina. From there it is conveyed by way of the optic nerve to the back of the brain and the sight center, where interpretation occurs.

Another aspect of the seeing art is in the physiological operation of the eyeball itself. As with all organs of the body, health of the eyes depends on three things: a constant flow of life force or nerve energy, proper nutrition, and the elimination of bodily wastes.

Your eyes do not possess the ability to obtain blood and nutrition but are to a large extent dependent on the overall condition of your body—the bloodstream, stomach and intestinal functions, kidneys, liver, lungs, and heart. Since the purity of your bloodstream greatly depends on the food you eat, it is obvious that your diet greatly affects your eyesight. The natural function of the eye is to see; thus, good vision is a natural occurrence unless it is obstructed by debris, denied its source of life supply, or saturated with poisonous matter.

The intake of too many medications injures the eyes. Many of our over-the-counter drugs contain mercury, quinine, arsenic, and other toxins. Some may contain morphine and other crystalline earthy substances that create uric acid. All of these substances are most injurious to eyes. They are equally poisonous to the entire body. If uric acid is deposited in the joints, one becomes arthritic. If deposited in mucous membranes or softer tissue in the body, the result may be cancer, tumors, ulcers, tuberculosis, or other diseases.

Like the tongue, the eye reflects the inner condition of the body. Many naturopaths diagnose the condition of the body by studying the eye. To them the eye is a complete map of the body's inner world. By studying the pupil or iris, they know instantly what disease may be developing within. Such a science is called *iridology*.

The Crystalline Lens

The crystalline lens, located just behind the iris, is a colorless, semisolid, transparent, biconvex disk suspended by ligaments. It is convex on both front and back surfaces, much like a magnifying glass. Its convexity varies constantly since it automatically adjusts for proper focusing on near or distant objects. It is composed of concentric layers, similar to an onion, between which run small lymph channels through which fluid passes into the substance of the lens.

When strain or tension is present, compression of the lens occurs, and the lymph fluid is blocked out. If blockage continues, the lens is denied its life force, and it becomes hard and dry. This dryness makes the lens slowly become opaque. If the strain and tension can be released, the pressure decreases, allowing the flow of fluid through the lymph glands—and the opaque cataract can sometimes be cleared away. Opaqueness also may result if the lymph fluid is filled with the wrong chemicals, placed there through wrong food, drugs, drink, numerous toxins.

The Eyes and the Brain Center

You do not actually see with your eyes, as has been explained. You see *with* your brain, with the sight center located toward the rear of the brain. The brain sight center dwells in total darkness, viewing the world *through* the eyes as channel-carriers of light rays. The pupil is merely a hole through which light rays travel to the retina at the rear of the eyeball, which in turn transmits images along the optic nerve to the visual center in the brain—upside down.

Instantaneously, your brain "develops" (photographically speaking) this image right side up. Only then do you see. The eye, then, is only an extension of your brain sight center. Just as the wizardry of a great pianist is achieved by the endless training of small muscles of the hands and fingers, so can the eye muscles, through very simple techniques, often be trained to achieve their ultimate purpose—perfect vision.

But remember, while the pianist can devote a lifetime to hand and finger dexterity, how many of us can devote hours each day toward the development of perfect vision?

CAUSES OF POOR EYESIGHT

The medical profession declares they know of no cause for poor eyesight, especially cataracts. They explain problems in strict medical terms, summing up the principal cause to be simply old age. But old age is not a cause. It's an effect.

At around age forty-five, most people find it difficult to read as they once did. Instead of beginning eye exercises for restoration, they go dutifully to the oculist for glasses. I did. But I also had the good sense to begin eye exercises and change my diet. Most people just get stronger and stronger glasses about every two years.

It is true that at middle age many muscles of the body begin to lose their tone, but this is not due to age. It is because years of no exercise and poor diet fill the muscles with toxins. The mind, responding, accepts the idea that one should walk less, dance less, swim less, play less tennis or golf. Just the opposite is true. The eyesight begins to blur because the eyes, being part of the body, are also filled with toxic substances and the muscles are losing their tone.

Many people readily adopt a program of walking, swimming, running, and so on as a means of keeping the body in shape. But they never once give thought to particular exercises to keep the eye in shape. They just buy glasses, which ensures that the eyes will forever remain out of shape. They accept the notion that at middle age the eyes "go bad." If we all would begin eye exercises just as we begin a walking or running program to keep the body young, the eyes would quickly adjust to the increased blood and pranic circulation, the increased muscle tone, the increased flow of moisturizing fluids. They would serve the soul for the full life term if properly treated.

In this section, we'll try to present what we believe to be major contributing factors toward poor eyesight, beginning with the most common of eyesight ailments: astigmatism.

Figure 4 shows us the three different eyeball shapes. The intricacies of the various common visual defects are easily explained on mechanical grounds. The three types are as follows:

The normal eye: Light rays correctly focus on the retina of the normal eye.

The nearsighted eye: If the oblique muscle becomes too tense, nearsightedness results. This eyeball is too long from front to back. Light rays focus in front of retina.

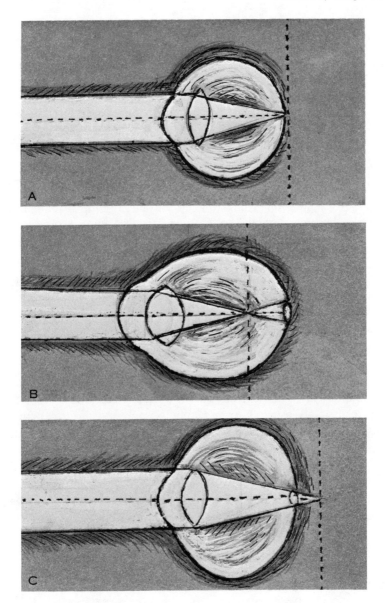

Figure 4. Eyeball shapes: a) in the normal eye, the light rays focus on the retina; b) in the nearsighted eye, light rays focus in front of the retina; and c) in the farsighted eye, light rays focus behind the retina.

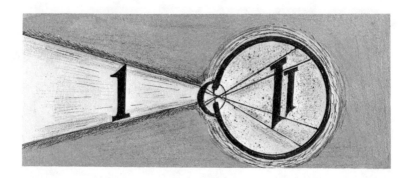

Figure 5. Astigmatism results when the tension of the oblique and recti muscles becomes unequal so that one group of muscles pulls more strongly than its opposite. The eyeball becomes lopsided by this unequal pressure, and blurred vision usually results.

The farsighted eye: If the recti muscles tighten into habitual tension, the light rays will focus behind the retina, causing farsightedness. This eyeball is too short from front to back.

Note especially the mechanical error that differentiates the nearsighted from the farsighted eye. Remember, too, the principle that all normal motions are good and strengthening for all eyes. Correct use of the eyes, plus proper exercise and diet, have been known to maintain or restore normal eye function regardless of the refractive fault.

When the tension of the oblique and recti muscles becomes unequal, one group of muscles pulls more strongly than its opposite set. The eyeball is therefore made lopsided by the unequal pressure, and astigmatism results. (See figure 5.)

Cataract

There are two major types of cataracts: *developmental* and *degenerative*. Developmental cataract is blamed on heredity or on nutritional or inflammatory disturbances. Degenerative cataract is usually associated with senile degenerative changes of various causes: radiation (including X-rays), trauma, diabetes, or exposure to toxic substances, such as drugs.

To be specific, there are several different types of cataracts:

1) *traumatic cataract*, caused by a perforating injury;

2) *irradiation cataract*, caused by exposure to certain rays;

3) *complicated cataract*, the result of various other ocular diseases;

4) *congenital cataract*, a condition with which one is born, usually arising from an impaired formation during fetal life; a malformation of the anterior chamber and a lack of contact of the lens with the cornea.

Cataract is an eye condition found far too often. What is not often found is its cause. It is usually related to old age, but cataracts often develop as early as the thirties, and in more recent years they have been found even in infancy and childhood. For every effect there must be a cause; generalized "old age" explains nothing. (The same is true for glaucoma.) Cataract has become very commonplace, now reaching epidemic proportions. Could our universal bad diet of recent years—the lack of proper vitamins, minerals, enzymes, riboflavin (B^2)—be to blame?

Most people believe that cataract is a film that grows over the eye and that the ophthalmic surgeon peels it off like a thin layer of offending tissue. This is not true.

Senile or degenerative cataract is the loss of transparency of the crystalline lens inside the eye just behind the pupil. An operation for cataracts means that the crystalline lens, which has lost is transparency, is removed from inside the eye. The clouding, or opacity, usually begins at one border of the lens and progresses slowly until the entire lens is covered, resulting in blindness.

Medical scientists say the cause of the opacity is unknown. Perhaps they seek a specific cause and fail to recognize the general causes. They seem to view the eye as separate and apart from the body, seeking a cause solely for the opacity that is slowly developing as a cloudy film on the lens of the eye. The only solution, according to medical science, is surgery—the removal of the entire crystalline lens—which means one must forever after wear suitable glasses or contact lenses, or be blind, because *removal of the cataractic crystalline lens results in blindness.* (We'll discus medical techniques in more depth in Part 4.)

The usual medical advice, once a cataract is discovered, is to "go home and wait until it matures" or "ripens," which is to say, "go home and wait until the lens is slowly covered with the cloudiness and you are nearly blind, after which surgery will be performed to remove the clouded lens." Usually no method of removing the cloudiness is ever offered— no mention of diet, exercise, or program of prevention, retardation, or correction. If you wish to practice preventive measures, you are usually left to develop your own program.

Usually both eyes are involved, one in advance of the other. The time required for cataracts to mature varies. Some develop fully in a few months; others very slowly, requiring many years of waiting—meaning many years of slowly going blind.

Although I may rouse the ire of most medical experts by offering methods and suggestions for arresting and even reabsorbing cataracts, I must confess that if total opacity has developed, surgery may be the only means of restoring sight. That is why it is imperative that preventive and curative measures be adopted as early as possible. Good eyesight can be perpetuated for a lifetime through proper diet, exercise, and as happy an attitude toward life as possible. Once cataracts have been diagnosed, however, curative measures —natural diet, exercise—must be begun at once, and the earlier the better.

Also, when cataracts are diagnosed, get a second opinion. Our government has released a report indicating that ophthalmic surgeons are now performing thousands of possibly unnecessary operations on the elderly, with Medicare paying most of the fee. Since 1965, when Medicare was first enacted, cataract operations have soared an incredible 146 percent. Twice as many operations are performed here as in Great Britain. So before submitting to any kind of surgical activities on your eyes, do get a second opinion from a surgeon you can trust.

In defense of doctors, it may be that the development of incredible new surgical techniques, such as lens implants, has led patients to demand the new operations rather than submit to the conventional methods. However, a second opinion is always justified in any ailment, and the desire for one should be understood.

When a doctor diagnoses cataracts and advises a patient to go home and wait for the cataract to ripen before surgery can be performed, it indicates that he or she can offer no program that will either stop the growth or cause the growth to be reabsorbed and disappear.

It means that the doctor assumes you will go right on living your chosen life-style, eating the foods and drinking the beverages that have contributed to the condition in the first place. It is unlikely that many ophthalmic surgeons have ever placed their patients on a nutritional program or suggested eye exercises that would offer improvement. Surgery means the total crystalline lens will be removed. The operation is called *surgical extraction of the eye lens.*

Once a ripe cataract develops in one eye, physicians often remove the lens in both eyes, even though the "good" eye has only the bare beginnings of a cataract. This enables the patient to adjust to the strong glasses or special contact lenses in both eyes simultaneously. This may or may not be a wise approach, depending on the patient's viewpoint.

Also, it is becoming popular now to proceed to the operation without waiting for cataracts to mature. There have been some remarkable scientific breakthroughs, which indicate that there are alternatives to waiting for "ripening." You can choose to have lens implants—which I'll tell you about in Part 4 of this book—or decide to change your life-style and opt for recovery of good eyesight through proper diet and exercise.

Nutritional Deficiencies and Cataract

Cataract can be said to be a nutritional disorder of the crystalline lens. Having no blood vessels, the crystalline lens must depend entirely for its nourishment on the aqueous or watery fluid that is continuously secreted and excreted. When the flow of the aqueous fluid is obstructed, the crystalline lens does not receive proper nourishment, thus losing its healthy optical transparency. When this happens, cataracts begin.

The aqueous fluid is secreted behind the iris, flowing through the pupil to fill the space between the iris and the cornea, the optically transparent front part of the eye. The rate of inflowing fluid is balanced by an outflowing secretion, which is accomplished by the aqueous fluid being reabsorbed into the blood. Problems develop when the rate of excretion is too slow. The inflowing aqueous fluid causes pressure buildup inside the eye, causing what is known as glaucoma. So cataracts result from an insufficient supply of aqueous fluid, whereas glaucoma results from too much of this fluid collecting in the internal space between the iris and the cornea. In a healthy eyeball there is a balanced flow of the aqueous fluid in the various areas.

Cataracts begin when the crystalline lens, isolated completely from the bloodstream, fails to receive nutrition via the aqueous humor. The aqueous humor receives its nutritional supply from the bloodstream and feeds the crystalline lens. When the aqueous humor fails to supply nutrients, the crystalline lens becomes cloudy and gradually loses its transparency. Thus, it may be clearly seen that nutrition could be a major contributing factor to cataracts and any other eye ailment.

The literature of most eye professionals readily recommends surgery, eyeglasses, contact lenses, drugs, and special treatments but rarely suggests the importance of proper nutrition. The holistic doctor, on the other hand, perceives the importance of nutrition, relief from stress, and the part played by emotions. Diet and stress are very prevalent causes of most eye troubles, and even the stress itself could be the result of improper nutrition.

I am by no means antimedicine or antisurgery; I believe in the development of modern approaches to save eyesight. I only suggest that nutrition and other natural methods be applied first. Then, if no results are obtained, surgery or other methods must be sought.

Since nutrition is a major factor contributing to cataracts and glaucoma, it would appear that certain foods may be involved in the development of cataracts. *Processed* dairy products—dairy products that have been pasteurized and chemically processed—seem to be among these. First of all, great thought should be given to the treatment of the cows producing most dairy milk. They are fed various antibiotics and given drugs and other chemicals to produce more milk. Processed dairy products are therefore loaded with preservatives and other chemical substances from innoculated cows. Raw milk, raw sweet butter, raw cream and raw cheese may be used in moderation; but pasteurized milk, processed cheeses, and other dairy foods have been found to be suspect in the development of cataracts.

When eaten in moderation, yogurt has beneficial qualities, but steady consumption of pasteurized yogurt is suspected of being directly linked to the development of cataracts. The high content of galactose (manufactured from milk sugar) in commercial yogurt is the culprit. Homemade natural yogurt is not included in this condemnation—only the popular commercial product available in supermarkets. Milk, from which yogurt is made, contains lactose, which breaks down into equal parts of glucose and galactose. A connection between galactose and the development of cataracts has been proved in tests with rats. Galactose in natural homemade yogurt is insufficient to cause damage. Its content is well below the dangerous levels found in the commercial product. In the commercial product the butterfat often has been removed, producing the low-fat product so much in demand.

Once the butterfat or cream has been removed, the consistency of the yogurt is watery and thin. To offset this weakness, manufacturers add skim milk powder, which contains a high percentage of milk sugar, or galactose. Home-made yogurt leaves the cream or butterfat intact. Use of whole milk in producing homemade yogurt reduces the galactose content, thereby reducing the danger of glaucoma and cataract. If you do buy commercially produced yogurt, choose the plain whole-milk product, not the low-fat one, and avoid the ones containing processed fruits.

Whey, that mysterious fluidic substance that accumulates in sour milk, is of inestimable value. Its mineral content is of extreme importance in nutrition required by the eyes. Although homemade yogurt seems to be supplied with whey, comercial yogurt is devoid of it. The whey content also has been removed from most processed cheeses.

Many people drink milk believing they obtain a valuable source of calcium. But pasteurized milk, because of its exposure to high heat, is not a good calcium source. Heat destroys the enzymes that make calcium assimilable by the body, but the harmful galactose in the milk sugar is by no means destroyed. Since pasteurization has destroyed the important enzymes to make the milk assimilable by the body, the galactose is extremely difficult to digest. The liver, unable to convert large amounts of galactose, often becomes enlarged. Jaundice could be the result, certainly an over-worked liver. Lack of calcium causes tension and muscle spasm contractions such as leg muscle cramps during the night.

During this process, what is happening to the eyes? The calcium so needed to avoid tension and muscle spasms is not being absorbed. Its lack creates muscle spasms, and even a slight muscle spasm in the eyes can cause serious damage. Lack of calcium also could be responsible for ongoing tension in the eye muscles, closing off the supply of healthy fluid and the circulation of the blood.

The assimilaton of calcium may be blocked if the body lacks its normal supply of vitamin D. That is why exposure to sunlight is important: to obtain vitamin D so that calcium may be absorbed. An excellent practice is a brisk early morning or late afternoon walk in the sunlight, when the ultraviolet rays are diminished. (Ultraviolet rays become excessive after 10:00 A.M. until around 4:00 P.M.) During the walk, the sunlight entering the eyes and cells of the body is of tremendous benefit. Walking itself is excellent exercise; together with exposure to pleasant sunlight, it is incomparable therapy.

Possibly the best way to keep the eyes healthy and avoid cataracts is to make sure your body is supplied with enzymes. The best natural source is live foods. This means daily salads of organically grown live foods (if organic fresh vegetables are available). All salad vegetables should be prewashed in apple cider vinegar water (about an ounce of vinegar to a gallon of water) to remove atmospheric pollutants. Of course, enzymes may be taken in pill form, but eating live foods is the best assurance of assimilation.

Cataracts, Old Age, and Enzymes

One reason cataracts develop in old age is that with the passage of years the body's supply of enzymes is depleted, and lack of enzymes could be the primary case of cataracts. It should be realized that cataracts, glaucoma, and other eye problems are not the result of weak eyes. The eyes have become weakened due to improper cell regeneration. Usually this regeneration can be traced to an improper diet, deficient in enzymes, which affects and weakens not only the eyes but the entire body. It is usually safe to say that when eye problems develop there are other health problems as well.

Every cell in the body is sustained by cell regeneration. Cells are constantly dying and being replaced. The channels for removing dead cells should obviously remain open and free-flowing. If the channels that remove the waste materials of the eyes become obstructed, then the ingathering debris and toxins, denied an exiting channel, will impair vision and create eye problems. A cataract develops when the crystalline lens has become damaged and obstructed because waste materials cannot flow freely from the eye, nor can proper nutrients flow in.

We have explained that cataract surgery means that the important crystalline lens is to be removed. Since one must ever after wear either contact lenses or a pair of strong, properly fitted glasses to substitute for the removed crystalline lens, it is extremely wise to be aware of nutritional importance before problems develop. Like every other cell, the cells of the eyes should be properly nourished and waste removed so that obstructions do not develop. Since it usually requires many years for cataracts to attain maturity, it seems reasonable that they can be diminished, held in abeyance, or completely disappear with exercise and diet—which would include natural remedies, such as herbs. And it is far better to adopt proper health and nutritional habits long before treatment becomes necessary.

I believe ordinary table salt contributes to cataracts. I suggest using sea salt, and that in moderation. Margarine contains many objectionable nutrients, including salt. Use sweet raw butter instead.

Causes of Cataract

1) Galactose from processed milk (not raw).

2) Lack of certain substances in the body, such as enzymes, vitamins, calcium and other minerals.

3) Poor circulation.

4) Continual strain, tension, and stress.

5) Lack of exercise.

6) Lack of sunlight.

7) Nitrates, nitrites, sorbitol, and other additives found in processed food.

8) Radiation from fluorescent lights, television, exposure to radar, leaking microwave ovens, smog, fallout from our atmosphere.

9) Overall bad diet—lack of raw live food, too many processed foods, sugar, salt, too much meat, too much fat, chocolate, caffeine.

Glaucoma

In a healthy eye there is a movement of a fluid that constantly bathes and nourishes the entire eye. Glaucoma results when this fluidic movement slows down because of obstructions in tiny canals inside the eyeball, creating pressure by the backed-up fluid, which gradually damages the retina and optic nerve. The fluid is filled with debris and toxins reflecting the same debris and toxins that flow through the bloodstream. If the canals allowing this toxic fluid to drain away become constricted, pressure inside the eye hardens the eyeball. If the pressure is not corrected, blindness could result. There are three principal types of glaucoma:

1) *Acute* (narrow angle), in which the blockage of the eye drainage comes suddenly, with no warning. It is usually accompanied by severe pain, redness and irritation, headaches, nausea, even vomiting. Usually an alarming reduction in vision occurs. Examination reveals dilation of the pupil.

2) *Chronic* (open angle), which occurs slowly and unnoticed. What *is* noticed is a gradual loss of field vision.

3) A secondary type caused by blockage, which in turn has been caused by infection, injury, or a possible tumor near the drainage canal.

Open-angle glaucoma is the most usual, the type that occurs without warning and without any obvious symptoms. Because there is seldom any pain or discomfort, it is suggested that the eyes be examined regularly—at least every two years. The only warning is an awareness of a gradual diminishing of field or peripheral vision, while the straight-ahead vision remains good. Usually one pays little attention to diminishing peripheral vision, but the slightest suspicion should send one for an eye examination. The blockage of the aqueous outflow channels is called *stenosis*.

Again, prevention, through proper nutrition and exercise, is the best possible measure to make sure the canals of the eyes remain open, flowing, and flexible. When the eye develops glaucoma, it is obvious that there must be similar blockages over the entire body, with the eyes symbolizing the most sensitive point. By preventing eye diseases one also may be preventing heart disease and high blood pressure.

When poor nutrition has been part of the life-style for many years, and glaucoma has resulted, frequently there is no solution except surgery—which is no solution at all. It only temporarily relieves the pressure. It is recognized that drugs, stress, worry, and even insomnia are factors causing glaucoma.

Another cause is arteriosclerosis, or hardening of the arteries—which is another way of saying a faulty diet. A malfunctioning pituitary gland also could be a factor, as well as disturbance of the autonomic nervous system. Glaucoma could result from lack of vitamin C. Glaucoma and cataract appear in persons accustomed to drinking large quantites of pasteurized milk. An incredibly high incidence of glaucoma is found among a religious sect in India called the Jains, who consume large quantities of pasteurized milk.

Coffee drinkers are also subject to glaucoma, it being well established that coffee—even caffeine-free—has a detrimental effect on the eyesight. Tobacco in any form—cigarettes, cigars, pipes—is known to be a cause of glaucoma, since tobacco constricts the blood vessels supplying the optic nerve with fluids and nutrition. Certain antispasmodic drugs also contribute, as well as steroid drugs.

Surgery usually consists of cutting a hole in the anterior chamber of the eyeball to allow drainage of the fluid. Even after successful surgery—meaning that the eyesight has been saved—prescription eyedrops are required to keep the pupils dilated. This treatment usually must persist the remainder of one's life. The use of drugs dropped into the eye is often an alternative to surgery, since these drops permit excess fluid to flow from the eyeball.

Various drugs are employed to treat glaucoma, the one most widely used being pilocarpine. It originally was produced by the leaves of a plant called *Pilocarpus microphyllus*, but it is now produced synthetically. It can have serious side effects—namely, nausea, vomiting, diarrhea, tachycardia, miosis, flushing, diaphoresis, and pulmonary edema, which could occur in patients with heart problems. Since both the treatment and the surgery are drastic measures, it would seem wise to begin now the proper regimen to avoid this unfortunate condition. Many naturopaths claim to have cured glaucoma through fasting, a diet of natural foods, and a good program of vitamins, minerals, and enzymes. Many naturopaths also report that an extended use of belladonna may cause glaucoma.

Dr. Som said that usually drugs containing iodides are prescribed for this disease, since they reduce the ocular pressure and thin the overly thickened cornea. But he prescribed the raw onion, which, cut close to the eye, causes watering and tears. Continued for only about a half minute, the natural iodides in the onion, causing the eyes to water and "cry," also reduce the ocular pressure and thin the thickened cornea. The tearing should not continue for more than a half minute, and the tears should be washed away with cold water immediately. Repeat the treatment three times a day in the beginning. Usually relief is experienced within six weeks. So said Dr. Som.

SYMPTOMS AND WARNING SIGNS

There are several obvious warning signs and symptoms of which one should be aware, any one of which could suggest glaucoma, cataract, or other eye problems:

1) *Blurred vision* is an early symptom and sign of cataract, but all who experience it are not necessarily such victims. Blurred, grayed, or blacked-out vision, especially when first wakening, could indicate inflammation of the retina. Blurred vision should send one quickly to an expert ophthalmologist for investigation. Blurred vision can be recognized through difficulty in seeing things as clearly as usual; necessity for holding objects closer to the eye; and needing a brighter light for reading.

2) Myopia (nearsightedness) may develop, meaning that one may not need reading glasses but may find it difficult to see at a distance.

3) Spots may appear, either dark or light.

4) Double vision may occur. Streetlights or the moon may appear double. Other objects may appear in a double outline. This could indicate hemorrhaging, a tumor, diabetes.

5) Frequent necessity for eyeglass changes.

6) Diminished vision, such as inability to clearly read signs on a bus, a street bench, newspaper ads. Such loss could indicate cataracts.

7) Inability to distinguish colors could indicate inflammation of the optic nerve.

8) Distorted vision, such as straight lines appearing crooked, could indicate a buildup of fluids inside the retina of the eye.

9) Vision through a red haze or streaks could signify bleeding inside the eye.

10) Loss of night vision could indicate problems with the optic nerve.

11) A change in your peripheral vision—such as when you look at someone's face but can't see the chest, or when a scene appears clear only in the center while the surrounding space seems dim, or if flashes cross your field of vision—could indicate glaucoma.

12) Persistent mucous discharge or excessive watering may suggest an infection or the presence of a foreign body.

13) Intense pain could indicate an infection or damage to the cornea through a foreign object, a scratch, or an injury.

14) Red eyes could indicate an infectious inflammation of the iris or acute glaucoma.

15) The appearance of halos around objects, especially lights, might indicate retinal problems.

Proper diet and exercise should prevent most or all these symptoms. But should they be obvious, do see your ophthalmologist for corrective measures. This book is not meant to suggest you avoid help from your doctor when such is indicated.

PART 2

THE METHODOLOGY OF
DR. WILLIAM BATES

Use your eyes! Live each day as though you may be stricken blind the next—and you will discover a world of wonder that you have been taking for granted, or have never seen at all!

—Helen Keller

THE BATES SYSTEM

Dr. William H. Bates was an oculist practicing in New York at the beginning of the 1900s. He prescribed glasses in the usual orthodox manner and performed surgery in the largest hospitals, such as Belmont and Columbia. But he had an intuitive feeling there was a better way to treat eyes. He inwardly rebelled against surgery, and felt that glasses were a crutch. He believed that with proper treatment surgery might be prevented.

When first beginning his practice, he accepted what was popularly accepted by the entire medical profession as the "Helmholtz theory of accomodation." This theory, elaborated by Dr. Herman Ludwig von Helmhotz between 1850 and 1895, stated that nearsightedness (difficulty seeing at a distance) and farsightedness (difficulty seeing near at hand) were caused by the shape of the crystalline lens. But Dr. Bates had a theory of his own. He discovered that even after removing lenses from the eyes, the eyes were still able to be taught accommodation at a near or far point. He proved his theory that the eye can adapt itself to varying distances just as it adapts to light and darkness. He claimed, and proved, that accommodation occurred by the *eye* changing the shape of the crystalline lens, and thereby the very shape of the eyeball itself. The eye accomplished this through using the extrinsic eye muscles, with their varying pull on the eyeball.

Since it was proved that the lens was not the chief factor of accommodation, Bates believed that eyesight failure in middle life was due to some change in these external muscles. These muscles almost completely surround the eyeball, and the contraction of certain of them lengthens the eyeball for near vision while others release for distant vision. He concluded that glasses destroyed the possibility of strengthening and correcting the function of these muscles, because the eye became "lazy," and did not do the work.

Most medical men and optometrists in this country refused—and still refuse—to accept Bates' findings. Medical theory is that the crystalline lens is the only means of accommodation, that accommodation to distance is accomplished by the pupil, by various changes in the lens, and by the curvature, axial thickness, and diameter of the lens. Dr. Bates holds that the shape of the eye, through the functions of the recti and oblique muscles, is altered to afford accommodation, just as the pupil automatically opens and closes to accommodate light and darkness.

Before he passed over, Dr. Bates trained teachers to carry on his work. The Bates Method is not a static thing, for teachers everywhere are constantly discovering additional techniques to correct eyesight. Bates teachers are found in many larger cities and in several countries.

In defense of the Helmholtz theory—that there is no cure for most eye problems except glasses—it must be said that glasses (including contact lenses) have certainly been a blessing for millions.

In praise of the Bates system, it has been proved over and over again that, for those willing to take the time and make the effort, there *is* a cure for eye difficulties—and there is prevention. So we must conclude that both systems work, depending on the person involved.

To accommodate all viewpoints, there should be in the office of every ophthalmologist a person qualified to teach a corrective program to those who prefer this approach. The patient should be asked: Do you wish glasses or would you prefer to be taught corrective methods?

Many would choose both. Many would ask for glasses until the corrective program slowly improved the eyesight—with the purchase of weaker rather than stronger glasses when indicated. But millions would prefer to walk into an office, have their eyes tested, and walk out with glasses or contacts, rather than give the time and effort necessary for correcting and perfecting their eyesight. The sad part is that so very many, not aware that there *is* a corrective program, meekly submit to glasses. My only criticism is that I believe they should be given a choice.

Both the Bates and the yogic systems recognize a connection between the muscles that surround the eyes and their focusing power. Four of these muscles are straight and two are oblique, as already stated. Because of their function, you can turn your eyes in any direction. Learning to use these muscles properly can correct common errors of vision such as nearsightedness and farsightedness. So says Dr. Bates.

THE THREE BASIC SECRETS

Dr. Bates stressed what he called the three basic secrets: central fixation, blinking, and shifting.

Central fixation: Bates claimed that the principal cause of strain, tension, and visual disorder was the habit of seeing too great an area of an object at one time. He retrained and reeducated his patients to look at—to focus on—only a small area of an object at a time, to achieve *central fixation.* He was attempting to train his patients to focus with and through the *fovea centralis,* the center of sight in the eye about which we have already told you.

Blinking: Another important function often neglected because of lack of awareness is that of blinking. A small gland called the *lacrimal* gland, under the outer portion of the upper lid, produces the fluid that keeps the eyes moist. Blinking stimulates the gland, causing the oily fluid to wash down over and into the eyeball. It not only acts as an antiseptic, cleansing and purifying the eyes, but it nourishes the cornea, which has no blood vessels. This important fluid flushes out foreign matter that may enter and damage the eye.

The average person is not conscious of how he or she blinks or how often. It's well to check your blink habits. As with all things, there is a right way and a wrong way. Nervous persons blink too hard and too constantly. The correct blink is the little, light, quick one. If you will practice a light fluttering blink consciously for a few moments each day it will soon become an unconscious habit. Here is your drill:

1) When you wake in the morning, blink ten light fluttery blinks, looking around the room as you do so.

2) Close your eyes a moment, open, ten more blinks, and close.

3) Continue the first morning until you have performed five sets of the ten blinks, fifty in all. The next morning add five more sets, one hundred in all. Each morning after that perform the ten sets of ten blinks.

These blinks, acting as lubricators for the eyes, can be repeated at any time during the day. Stimulating the tear ducts, blinking keeps the eyes moist. Dryness of the eyeballs can cause serious problems.

Blinking also breaks the destructive stare. Staring, strained eyes seldom blink properly. Correct blinking also prepares the eyes to accept and tolerate more light. If you blink properly, you will find less tendency to squint your eyes against the bright light.

4) After the hundred blinks, squeeze the eyes tightly, then open them wide. Repeat three times only.

Shifting: Shifting is what has just been mentioned—allowing the eyes to shift from point to point when viewing an object. Focus your vision on a small area of an object, then blink, then shift your seeing to another point.

1) Fixation (focus on a small area)

2) Blink (a light, quick, fluttery blink)

3) Shift (pass with great speed from area to area of the object viewed)

Let's say you are looking directly into someone's face. Don't stare. Look first at the point between the eyebrows. Blink, then shift to the right eye, then the left. Then drop the focus to the lips, back up to the forehead, and complete the circuit to the eyes again.

The shift becomes habitual. This same procedure should be practiced each time you view any object.

THE EXERCISES

In addition to the blinking and shifting techniques, Dr. Bates offered certain exercises he felt would restore the troubled eye to normalcy. They include, most significantly, palming and sunning among the exercises that follow.

Palming

This marvelously simple method was first advocated by Dr. Bates more than fifty years ago and is still helping people. He describes the advantages of palming in his book *Perfect Sight Without Glasses*,[1] in which he provides case histories of people who were able to reverse eye ailments through this procedure.

Palming is a rest period for your eyes. It should be made the time of greatest mental relaxation. As with everything in

---

[1]William H. Bates, *Perfect Sight Without Glasses*, (New York: Central Fixation Publishing, 1920).

life, the eyes relate to the dualities of Earth—the opposites of dark and light. Healthy eyes require both dark and light, rest and activity. When your eyes are open, they are saturated with light. When they are closed and darkened, the retina and optic nerves absorb the light recently bathing the tissues. True black appears to "palmed" eyes only when your eyes and mind are relaxed. Thus, you may need to palm for a day, a week, or a month before you begin to see true black.

There is purple pigment in the retina called *visual purple.* This is used in night driving, for example. Light tends to absorb this element, but palming restores it. If you are having difficulty with night vision, try palming.

It is always good to palm the eyes after exposure to the sun. (See "Sunning" on page 50.) If you sun for five to ten minutes, then practice palming for ten to twenty minutes. Make this a general rule. If you are exiting into the sun, pause a moment to deliberately expose your eyes. It may be impossible to palm immediately afterward, but do close your eyes for the duration of a long breath before proceding on your way.

There is no set rule or time for palming. Any time is a good time. Much depends on the time you can give it, your occupation, and other factors considered. If possible, practice two or three palming intervals during the day. Even brief practice will benefit your eyes greatly. If one fifteen-minute period is impossible, take three five-minute intervals. Five minutes will help if that is all the time you have. These suggestions are for so-called normal eyes. If you are experiencing visual difficulty, definite times for palming are imperative.

Eyes with problems, including circulatory or similar difficulties, should be given as much time as possible for palming. Such eyes—indeed the entire body—need much relaxation. Any debilitating illness, such as influenza, will lower the vitality of the eyes. Palming will be of inestimable value in restoring normalcy. After an illness the eyes, being weakened, should not be strained with too much visual work, such as reading. The more time given to palming, the more quickly their normal strength will be restored.

Palming may be the only time your eyes have total rest. Eyes do not necessarily rest during sleep. When you reach the age of responsibility, you have simultaneously attained the age of worry—and the potential for night strain. Look at your eyes in the morning, and you will often see tired eyes even after a night's sleep.

If palming is correctly done, all tension is released. The darkness rests and reenergizes. A pranic healing magnetism flows from your hands into your eyes. The warmth increases the circulation. Fifty-four times a second the eyes are washed by a specialized bloodstream. This is doubled during palming. The retinal nerves are nourished, venous blood carries away the poisons in the eye, and the arterial blood brings fresh nourishment. The importance of this increased blood and life-force circulation cannot be overemphasized. It is extremely beneficial for the entire body. The usual comment after palming is "I feel rested all over." Also, if the long swing is performed at bedtime, the eyes are relaxed for a nights sleep, and insomnia frequently is overcome.

When the eyes are healthy, they act as channels through which pranic light and life force from the very atmosphere flow into and vitalize all the body cells. The hands are also such channels. Combining the two channels through palming is doubly effective for flooding body cells with high-voltage pranic light. To sit in a dark room with your eyes closed is not a substitute for palming. Neither is placing a dark cloth over your eyes. Neither provides the incomparable power of contact with human hands.

If you are intensely nervous, impatient, or high strung, early efforts at palming may be difficult. Performing a few active-relaxing drills first may be helpful. (See "Swings and Drills.") If you begin to feel restless during palming, stop at once and perform more active-relaxing drills. You should never try to force passive relaxation. That would defeat the entire purpose.

The Technique

First, sit in a comfortable position. Your whole physical body should be relaxed as well as your eyes. You may use one of several methods for supporting your elbows. One is to hold an object such as a wedge-shaped pillow on your lap, resting your elbows on it, or you can rest your elbows on a table. You may prefer to lie on your back if your arms can remain comfortable. Whichever method is used, be sure your neck is in a straight line with your spine, pushing your head neither forward nor backward.

Rub your hands briskly together before placing them over your eyes, increasing their circulation and stimulating the flow of prana through them. Visualize them as highly charged "generators" through which tremendous power is flowing—a stream of pure white light.

Before placing your hands over your eyes, lift your eyebrows so that, while palming, the weight of your brows is lifted from your eyes. This nourishes nerves around your eyes and removes strain in any eye muscles.

Form your hands into hollow cups and place the cupped palms over your eyes as shown in figure 6. The bony part of your hands, just above the wrist, should rest on your cheekbones. With your fingers crossed over the top of your nose, resting lightly against your forehead, your cupped hands will fit nicely over your eyes and exclude all light. There should be no feeling of weight or pressure on your eyes.

Open your eyes only once to be sure all light is excluded. If slits of light appear, adjust your hands until there is total darkness, then close your eyes lightly. With practice you will soon be able to place your hands correctly.

What should you do while you palm? First of all, try mental pictures—guided imagery. There is a right way and a wrong way. Remember, you are using your eyes as paintbrushes, not staring at any object trying to see the whole

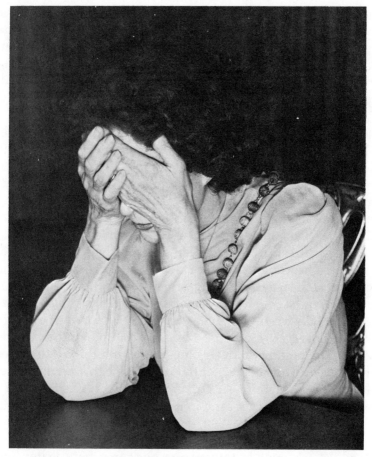

Figure 6. The technique of Palming.

picture at once. Staring can happen while palming. Avoid it by visualizing active mental pictures.

Think of a cool darkness. If at first there seem to be gray foglike streaks of color, ignore them. Do not focus on them, wondering what they are. They are caused by eye strain and tension in most cases and will vanish as you become relaxed and interested in your mental pictures. Try to create a field of pure darkness on which to draw your pictures.

Always draw your scenes from the memory of some happy time. Recall a birthday party you especially enjoyed.

Picture the guests coming into the room. See them moving toward you with gaily wrapped gifts. Imagine your hands moving out (really watch their movement) to receive them. See yourself untying the ribbon, tearing the paper, opening the package. See whatever gift comes most easily to mind. Look at it detail by detail—remember, eyes are paintbrushes. Take another gift.

Recall more happy happenings. Picnics or a circus parade. Thanksgiving. A remembered Christmas—white snow, the sleigh, the group around the laden table, the fireplace. Go to the attic and open a trunk of beloved memories. Take out precious objects you loved in the past years, each one stirring memories of a happy event, painted by your eyes on a mental canvas. What happy images to create while palming!

See yourself near the ocean. You are lying on the sand. The sun is warm on your face. A soft, cool breeze carries the scent of a nearby flowering shrub. Now the scent of salt water. Breathe deeply and remember the sharp, tangy aroma.

Mentally open your eyes—not actually, for your eyes are always closed as you palm. Mentally sit up and look at the water. The ocean is a lovely blue-green with the white waves breaking on the shore. Gently at first. Then they increase. Here comes a big one—it strikes the shore. It recedes with a swish, leaving the wet sand in its wake, with bits of kelp and seashell.

Let your eyes drift out over the water. A sailboat is there. Watch it glide toward the horizon where water and sky merge in a soft lavender. Two seagulls nearby attract your attention, both diving for the same fish. The victorious one makes off with it. The other soars silently over the water, rising to the sky like a winged, slow-moving rocket. It vanishes, leaving your mental canvas dark again.

Stretch and inhale deeply. Then totally relax to complete your palming. You may be almost asleep! In these scenes, remember the feel of things—the warm sand trickling through your fingers, the rough shell of the peanut, the tingle of the ocean spray, the sound of the gulls, the waves. Such vivid visualization increases the activity of all of your senses. All senses function through the same ganglion network. It is well to increase their ability to maximum performance. What helps one helps the others.

It is advisable to include black and white mental pictures in your imagery. Such "visioning" aids the eyes to see black print on a white page. Example: a lawn covered with white snow, soft and blue-white in the shade. A black Scotty dog chasing a ball, which can be of any color. As he runs he breaks the snow. See his small black footprints. Here comes a little girl, tossing the ball. She is wearing a red snowsuit with a hood. Watch the black dog run across the white snow after the ball. She builds a snowman. He is wearing a black hat. Big black buttons adorn his white front. He holds a black cane. The snowman melts, leaving a blank canvas.

Picture a beautiful black velvet dress. Feel it. Nothing quite like the feel of velvet. Watch the motion of your hands as you unwrap a florist's box. Take from it a white gardenia, carnation, or rose. Smell it! Remember the aroma. Feel the petals, the crisp leaves. Pin the white flower on the black dress. What a beautiful contrast, white on black. How easy to see. Now reverse the picture. Pin a black velvet rose on a white velvet dress.

For those who find this mental picturing difficult or tiring, select easier choices. Think of a blackboard with soft white chalk. You print a large capital *A* on it. Watch your hand erase it. Print a *B, C, D*, erasing each as you draw the next. Go through the alphabet, keeping the letters large.

These drills also may be practiced when you retire, to relax your body and enter mental tranquility. When your body and mind are both tranquil, sleep can't be far behind.

Palming may be done mentally. With practice, you can memorize the feel of your palming hands—soft, relaxed, warm over your eyes—and the gentle darkness. While waiting for an appointment or traveling on a bus, you may think, "If I could only spend this wasted time palming." You can, mentally, and receive much help and relaxation.

Have you ever visited a fair, museum, or art gallery only to have the visit spoiled with aching feet? You wondered why, since your shoes were comfortable and you really hadn't walked very much. It could be your eyes. Yes, straining your eyes can affect your feet! There are close nerve connections between the two. By looking intently, trying to see so much, you have unconsciously been staring. Your eyes have transferred their discomfort and tension to your feet. If possible, find a quiet spot, sit down for a few moments and palm mentally or physically. It is incredible how quickly you can sally forth again, totally regenerated.

Learn to make palming one of your happiest habits. You will be using one of the greatest secrets of health for your eyes and youth for your body. Visualizing while palming also unfolds the psychic faculty of clairvoyance.

Sunning

The sun is certainly the physical light of the world. And light is the secret of all life. It was God's edict—*Let there be Light*—that started the whole cosmic drama. Made in the image of God, the soul also needs light. If the eyes truly are the windows of the soul, then the eyes certainly need light to remain a pure and perfect window.

Light, especially sunlight, is God's method of healing the body, even through the eyes. Light flowing into and through the eyes stimulates brain cells and glands; and obviously, whatever affects the brain, making it more receptive to mind/thought power, affects the whole body with its cells and glands. Sunlight, entering the eyeball gateway, stimulates first the pituitary/pineal glands, and their "quickening" stimulates the whole being through the endocrine glandular system, an oxygenized, purified bloodstream, and newborn body cells.

Working with light is one of the most important phases in establishing health for the eyes, for relaxation and for revitalizing the retinal nerves. Too many eyes are supersensitive to light. In most cases this supersensitivity is caused by fear of light rather than the light itself. People are brainwashed. "Don't let that light shine in your eyes." In a room they are afraid to sit facing the light from a window, even when the light is dimly filtered in through trees. Venetian blinds or heavy drapes are drawn to spare the eyes from the light.

It is a common sight to see dark glasses worn in a lecture hall or other public gatherings even at night. What started as a senseless fad a few years ago has today grown, for many, into a necessity. In a recent book a top model warns never to be caught in the sun without dark glasses because exposure will damage the eyes! What nonsense! How did we ever manage all these millions of years before some Hollywood starlet decided to don dark glasses as a part of her mystique?

To wear dark glasses when an ophthalmologist has not prescribed them for a special purpose is foolish. It is true that occasionally a special eye problem requires temporary shielding. But usually there is no necessity for them. In fact, they are harmful. Did God make the eye so delicate an organ that, to function and fulfill its purpose, it must be shielded artificially from light? Actually, the eye is the one organ in the body constructed by God and by nature to absorb light into itself. And maintaining healthy eyes calls for normal exposure to sunlight. Light is required to stimulate the nerves of the retina.

It is feared the infrared rays from the sun (rays that warm us and supply heat to the Earth) and the ultraviolet rays (that tan us) will damage the eyes. Nature has designed our bony eye pockets to jut out above our eyes to protect them from the rays of very intense light energy. Our hairy eyebrows also act as natural shields, not only from the sun but from the rain.

Actually it is the "upward reflection" of intense sunshine on manmade materials such as flagstones and cement that causes unpleasant glare against which the pupils of the eyes contract, become strained, and need shielding. The only time dark glasses are ever advised is during a temporary exposure to this upward reflection, such as a long drive on a cement road during intense summer heat. Outdoor workmen such as telephone linemen and construction workers may be justified in wearing dark glasses during the midday hours of intense summer heat. But most do not, and they seem to fare all right. They are so busily moving and working, their eyes are seldom exposed to direct infrared or ultraviolet rays.

The only people who are truly justified in wearing dark glasses would be people who fish or enjoy being out on the water who are exposed to reflective sun glare; drivers whose jobs expose them to glare from cemented streets; police officers, people who work outdoors, such as construction workers, exposed to midday glare on bright objects; beach people, such as lifeguards, who need protection from sand and water glare; skiers and ski instructors, when the snow reflects sun glare.

Habitual use of dark glasses causes far more damage than exposure to sunlight. In addition to the damage already mentioned, their use will diminish your natural ability of 100 percent color perception.

Sunshine is the one great stimulator of the optic nerve. It is also needed to relax tense muscles. Brainwashed people, taught to fear light, immediately become tense at the least exposure, reacting against it. They instinctively reach for their dark glasses or draw the shades. Many people, tensed with the fear of the light, even feel pain in their eyes when passing from a darkened room into the outdoor sun, further convinced the sun is harmful and damaging unless the eyes are protected. It is certainly true that when shielded long enough, the eyes become so weakened that light will indeed bring pain. *The lack of light, caused by too much shielding, has caused damage to the optic nerve, and such a weakened nerve will certainly react to sudden exposure.*

Following such damage, eyes can and should be corrected by gradual training and a rational approach to the light problem. Once you fully understand that the eye was given to you for the use of light, that the sun is the eye's best medicine, that the eye is indeed the greatest channel for bringing light and life force into the body *and* soul, you have taken the first great step in overcoming photophobia, or fear of light. Reeducating the mind and eyes to light must be taken in small steps, gradually overcoming the fear as you grasp the truth of it. Each step will give you a sense of freedom and well-being.

Let us suppose you are going from soft indoor lighting into your garden. Instead of rushing headlong into the bright light, pause in the doorway a moment with your eyes closed. Allow the brighter light to filter through your closed lids. Raise your eyebrows to thin out the little folds over the lids. This will prevent squeezing the lids tight and tensing against the light.

Now step out into direct sunlight, still with closed eyes. Swing your head slightly from side to side, keeping your eyes focused downward behind the closed lids. Expose your eyes one at a time with the swinging. You have taken your first small step.

Open your eyes slowly, still looking down and away from the sun, facing shade if possible. Do not face a glare on a wall or on a walk. If there is such a glare, look away from it but do not fear it. Remember, fear tenses the eyes. Stay in the sunlight only a brief time. If you have been accustomed to dark glasses over a long period of time, alternate between wearing and not wearing them, especially if a longer exposure is necessary. Next time, remain longer without the glasses. As your eyes grow stronger, discard the dark glasses altogether except when driving a car headed directly into the glaring sun or when exposed to beach sand reflection, snow glare, or reflected bright midday sun. There *are* special occasions when care should be taken.

If you are driving a car and are accustomed to dark glasses, take no chances. Let that be the last place to do without them, and then only as you become accustomed to going without them in comfort at all other times. This is important for your safety and the safety of others. Use common sense in all things.

After you have first taken the light on closed lids and the ordinary daylight in a relaxed way, you are ready for the next step, the sun. The sun! What would life be without it! How sickly the plant kingdom would soon become if there were no sun. Flowers turn their faces to the sun. Birds perched on telephone wires face the sun to sing. Children at play look fearlessly into the sky. Heads are often thrown back for momentary direct exposure. The child is not afraid. It is later that fear of light comes, when a well-meaning parent warns that eyes should be protected from "too strong sunlight." Dark glasses will be obtained, and the ritual of keeping out all the health-giving, sight-building benefits of the sun is begun. If sunlight is so damaging, isn't it strange that the eyes of *all* children aren't affected? Their constant movement during childhood play tends to prevent damaging exposure.

Babies too young to walk and move about *should* be protected from direct sunlight in the eyes. In baby carriages the infant should never be allowed to lie on its back looking up at bright sunshine. The face should always be shielded by a canopy. Actually, an infant should never be too long exposed to ultraviolet rays. Once a child begins to run about, the upright positon offers natural shielding.

Adults who insist on lying face up in direct sunlight for suntanning at midday *should* wear dark glasses. Such direct exposure to ultraviolet rays could be harmful. They also should be aware that these midday rays penetrate even dark glasses and closed lids, damaging the eyes. Eyes should *never* be directly exposed to a hot midday sun for extended periods. Exposure is safe until 10:00 in the morning and after 4:00 in the afternoon. The rays are dangerous only during the midday hours.

There is a right technique for taking the sun, and when it is used, no damage of any kind occurs. Instead, the eyes gradually become accustomed to the brightness—just as they were in childhood—and benefit by improved vision and a healthy optic nerve and retina.

The Technique

First step: Select a clear, bright day for your first sun practice. Sun shining through haze or smog is hard for all eyes;

even eyes conditioned to the sun are inclined to squint against such a light. So select a day when the sun is clear and bright.

With eyes *closed*, focus downward behind the closed lids. Lower your head. Step into the sunlight. Begin swinging your head in easy rhythm from side to side, gradually raising your head. Continue the swing until you are swinging across the face of the sun. Feel as though the sun were passing your face. This will give you a sense of motion necessary for loosening your eyes.

In all head swings turn your head from shoulder to shoulder. Repeat several times. If the light seems too sharp even with your eyes closed, swing across the bright sky near the sun for a few moments. Do not hold your breath. Breathe easily and rhythmically.

Now begin to swing your entire body instead of just your head. Lock your arms behind you, your right hand grasping your left forearm, and swing in a side-to-side arc, as in the Long Swing.

Remember to close your eyes lightly with your brows lifted. Before long you will feel a sense of ease and relaxation. Never allow your eyes to squint during your sunning or at any other time. Keep your face serene, never furrowed or frowning. Nothing will impair vision more quickly than frowning. It is often just a habit and one that can be broken with a little thought. Lift your brows and think looseness of the lids and muscles. Stay swinging in the sun only a few moments in the beginning. Gradually lengthen the time to ten or fifteen minutes if possible.

Most people do not have eyes nearly as large as they are meant to be because of squinting. Nothing will help to overcome this more than being able to handle light and sun with ease. Frequently ask yourself, "Am I squinting?" Release, release, release those muscles. *Think serenity. Always, at all times.*

Take the second step only after mastering the first one. Always begin each sunning with Step 1. This warms the eyes. Now proceed to Step 2.

Second Step in Sun Work

Cover one eye with the cup of one hand as in palming, closing out all light. With a head swing or body swing, blink rapidly and sweep the open, exposed eye back and forth three or four times across the sun as shown in figure 7. It is important that you swing your head and that you blink. *Never stare into the sun!* After one eye is sunned in the manner described, place a palm over the other eye, open and blink the exposed eye, repeating the drill. Always turn your head; always blink; never stare.

The sun's brightness will be greatly reduced by sunning one eye at a time. After long experience and practice, some people blink across the sun with both eyes at a time.

If your eyes water, good. Exposure to sun rays opens the tear ducts—with great benefits. Tears are nature's way of washing and purifying the eyes. They also release congested sinuses. Tear ducts spread moisture over the surface of the eye. The natural tear contains a strong chemical. Scientists have said that one tablespoon of tear solution equals many gallons of salt water. So tears are powerful against germs that might affect the eye. If the eye waters through healthy stimulation, only good can result. It is when the tear ducts do *not* function that trouble begins. If at first there seem to be afterimages of lingering spots of light, they soon disappear after a brief palming. This sunning and palming will relieve muscle spasms.

Always be reasonable in the use of the sun. Your face cannot and should not be too long exposed. Anytime the face feels hot, it is time to stop the practice. Several short practices a day are better than too long at a time. If you wish, sit on a lawn chair and, leaning your head back, move it gently from side to side, letting the sun play on the closed lids. Then practice the second step with each eye, followed by some palming, either in the sun or in the shade.

When you have practiced this sunning a few times, you will never again put on dark glasses (with the exceptions listed above). Your eyes will have grown accustomed to the

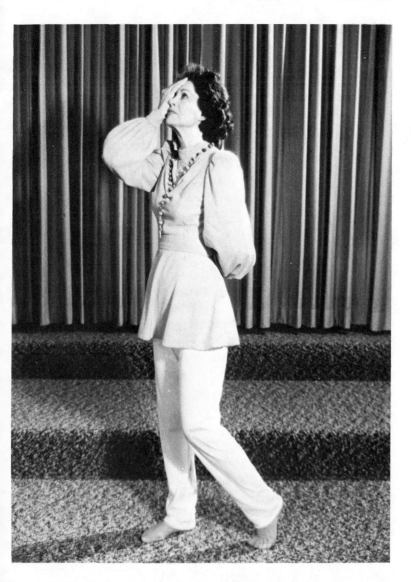

Figure 7. Sunning. Cover one eye with the palm of one hand and open the other eye to swing across the sun, blinking. Now change hands, open and expose the other eye, blinking repeatedly and swinging the body. After long practice, you can blink across the sun with both eyes open.

light. People who say they have always suffered from the light soon learn to love it. If at first there is any discomfort, practice for a longer time with the closed eyes directed toward the bright sky and not the sun itself, then blink across that brightness. Check the squint, for discomfort or pain could be caused by that alone by shutting off free circulation.

Follow these rules and only good can be the result. It bears repeating that the sun is God's best medicine for the eyes. Well-sunned eyes are bright and shining. They reflect an inner light. Bright eyes are *always* light eyes.

Common Sense and Sunlight

Most believe it is never wise to look directly into the sun deliberately. Yet many naturalists and yogis *do* face the rising sun at dawn, with apparent benefits to the eyes. However, white light reflected by snowclad areas can cause snow blindness, which is usually only temporary. Eyes should be shielded. The reflection of the sun's rays on a large rippling body of water or the smooth surface of the sea can produce sun blindness, which can be permanent. Each ripple constitutes a concave mirror that collects the heat rays from the sun and reflects them into the eyes. Common sense dictates shielding the eyes with dark glasses.

Eclipses of the sun subject the eye to a dangerous overdose of heat rays and should never be observed, even for a second, without the use of specially prepared glass or dark glasses. We have already said direct exposure during midday hours should be avoided. Shielding is wise to prevent damage from ultraviolet rays.

Sunning with an Electric Light

Sunning may be done indoors when weather does not permit outdoors. It requires preparation. Rig a light pole that can be moved from place to place with a 150-watt incandescent light bulb and a light reflector. Indoor sunning is then done as follows:

1) Sit 3 feet from the pole containing the 150-watt light bulb.

2) Eyes should be closed, feet flat on the floor.

3) With the full light on your face, turn your head slowly from side to side up to 10 minutes.

4) After 10 minutes, move 2 feet from light.

5) After practicing thus for a few days, place the 150-watt light bulb in the reflector and repeat the drill (sit farther away and use less wattage if uncomfortable).

6) Swing your head from side to side, eyes closed, for only 4 minutes.

Palm from 5 to 20 minutes following this indoor sunning. Then graduate to performing the entire technique with open eyes.

Alternative Method

Dr. Som suggested the following method for sunning:

1) Look at the sun with closed eyes for 1 minute the first day.

2) Look at the sun with closed eyes for 2 minutes the next day.

3) Repeat for 3 minutes the third day.

4) Rest a day.

5) Start again with 1 minute as before.

6) Palm after each sunning.

BATES DRILLS AND SWINGS

One of the things most necessary for those with tension, in both the eyes and the body, is to learn to relax more; learn to release body as well as eye muscles. As the muscles relax, the eyes learn to shift. Simultaneously, the little fovea accelerates its delayed movement, caused by tension. It gradually resumes its normal 70-times-a-second shift. This close relationship between eyes and mind was described in the previous section. Eye difficulties always result from lack of coordination between eyes and mind. Therefore, one major purpose of the swings and drills that follow in this section is to restore this necessary coordination.

There must be a mental awareness of looseness and released eye muscles. For example, when you close your eyes, close them lightly. Never clench them. Be constantly aware of the easy look. To many, just closing the eyes means tension. Their normal closing is so tight, they can see the pressure all around the eye. Instead, you should gently and easily close the lids over the eyeball. Feel them lightly laid over the eyes like rose petals, not as chunks of coal. Thinking softness and looseness, accompanied by a slight raising of the brows, lifting weight from the eyes, will be of great benefit in the first steps of relaxation.

As we grow older, our eyes tend to become smaller. Gone is the wide, open look of childhood. This is because the eyebrow muscles, having lost their tone, allow loose skin to settle over the eyes. Try consciously lifting the brows and massaging under them for a few moments with the thumb. You'll find the muscles becoming stronger and able to hold the eyebrows where they belong. Many times a day think "brows up." Before long, you'll be surprised to discover that when you think "brows up," they are already up.

As you plan a program of health for your eyes, it is imperative to establish right habits. After consciously practicing lightly closing and lifting your brows, you soon lose all tendency to clamp and padlock the lids. Remember, learn to "look easy," feel relaxation all around the eye, think looseness, *think serenity*, and do not squint.

Important! *Always* remove your glasses and contact lenses for the drills that follow. Even though you think you cannot see without them, you will be surprised how much you will see after the first palming–sunning. All sunning, even if you just face the sun for a moment, *must* be done without glasses or contacts. And this is what you must fully understand: *The principal purpose of exercising the eyes is to restore movement deep within the eye*, the action and relaxation of tension in and around the fovea.

The Elephant Sway

This exercise, shown in figure 8, on page 62, is so easy and simple! Just stand with your feet comfortably apart. Begin to sway from side to side, shifting your weight from one foot to the other with a rhythmic movement. Let your eyes follow the swaying, back and forth. Let them look at distant scenes. Outside landscapes will seem to move in the opposite direction. Or sway before a window with up-and-down bars or grillwork. As you sway, don't focus on the bars, just let them sway in the opposite direction to your own.

This simple practice trains the eyes to shift. It also stimulates circulation in the head. It often will cause "watering," which cleanses the eye. Don't sway from hip to hip; let your entire body move with the swing. Think of the elephant as he swings his trunk, easily, lazily back and forth. Practice this swing during any waiting period, such as waiting for an elevator, or on the street waiting for a bus. If you wish, fold your arms and hands behind you as described under "The Long Swing."

Go from the Elephant Sway into the Long Swing.

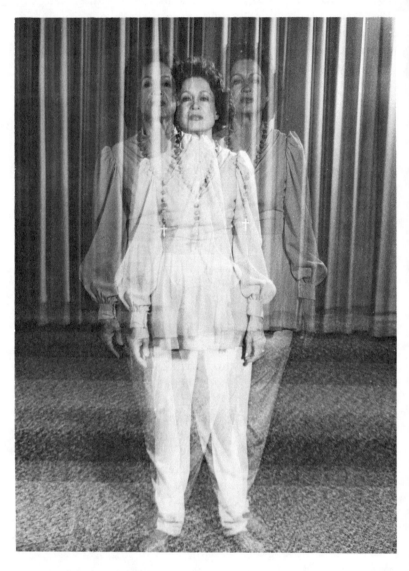

Figure 8. The Elephant Sway. Stand with feet comfortably apart. Begin swaying from side to side, shifting weight from one foot to the other. Be sure eyes follow the swaying, looking at distant scenes.

The Long Swing

A drill of major importance is the Long Swing shown in figure 9 on page 64. There are several reasons why this exercise is so important—its swinging motion starts the shift of the fovea, the 70-times-a-second shift deep in the eye; it eases tension in the spine, acting somewhat like a spinal massage; it loosens and relaxes the head and neck; it releases and stimulates the long body muscles; it balances the flow of nerve systems to calm that restless feeling a nervous person sometimes experiences. After performing this swing, it is often easier to relax and palm. The steps are as follows:

1) Stand with your feet about 10 or 12 inches apart, not too far for ease nor too close for steadiness. Avoid high heels; choose low heels, flats, or wedges or stand barefoot for strengthening the arches.

2) Allow your arms to fall easily at your sides, then forget them. They will swing in a natural pendulum motion as you sway your body. You may prefer to fold them across your back, the right hand grasping the left forearm.

3) Shift your weight from one foot to the other as you go into a swing, turning from side to side. For example, as you turn right, lift your left heel, giving a little push to the right with the toes—similar to a golf stance.

4) Turn your head and shoulders as you swing, keeping your eyes parallel with your nose, about half open in a dreamy way. Select a site on each wall on a level with your eyes. I choose a picture of Jesus hanging on a wall in my bedroom. I stand sideways to the picture. On each swing, I look directly into the Master's eyes for a split second. Just a notion of mine. Swing your full body with your shoulders paralleling the walls.

Never practice this drill in a dark room or with closed eyes. This could cause dizziness. Do not allow your eyes to

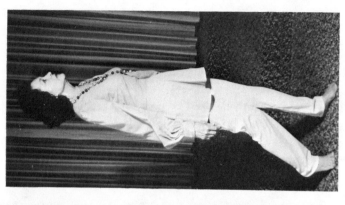
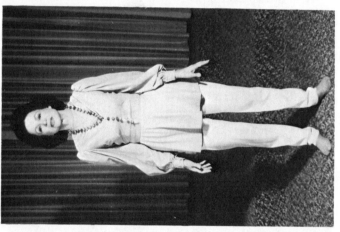
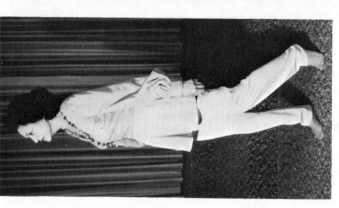

Figure 9. The Long Swing. Stand with feet comfortably apart, arms at the side or folded behind your back. Shift weight from one foot to the other, turning the body to parallel your shoulders with the walls in the room. Keep your eyes parallel with your nose.

roam upward, then down and around the room. This could cause severe headache. Do not thrash your body as you swing, but establish a rhythm.

5) Swing for 60 counts, the number required to bring relaxation. You will feel the stiffness of your body letting go. Add 40 more for good measure, and you will have a perfect relaxation drill. This should take about 10 minutes. As you swing, the objects in the room should seem to be moving in the opposite direction. Be sure your neck and shoulders are relaxed, your arms swaying gently with your body rhythm or folded behind you. Do not let your eyes pause on any object as you turn your head and body. Keep eyes and nose parallel.

If you have a record player, select a waltz, or hum a tune, swinging to its rhythm. If performed the last thing at night, this exercise will induce sleep and insure perfect fovea relaxation during the night. If done the first thing in the morning, it will start your day with eyes freely moving and shifting. This method, purely for relaxation and movement, prevents pressures and imbalances that produce cataracts and glaucoma. Pregnant women will find this swing of great value for relaxing tense muscles, especially during hours of labor. Tension is the principal cause of pain. This Long Swing is excellent to release tension and relax all muscles.

Short Swings

The foregoing drills are large-movement drills. Dr. Bates has said, "The shorter the shift the greater the relaxation," meaning, if you can shift your eyes a very short distance and get a small object moving in the opposite direction, there will be even greater relaxation. Try the following:

1) Stand about 6 feet in front of an open doorway. Take the same position as for the Long Swing.

2) Swing your eyes from one side of the door frame to the other, possibly with a slight body shift. The room beyond the

door should then seem to be moving in the opposite direction. Remember the principles: eyes parallel to nose, head and body moving in the same direction.

3) After you have achieved this sense of motion, point a finger at the lower left of door frame. Watch your finger as it travels from the lower door frame up the side to the upper corner, turn the corner square, eyes following finger across the top and down the other side, then across the bottom to left corner again. Repeat several times, then reverse the movement, going from right to left.

4) Repeat several times, then drop your finger and continue, letting your eyes follow through alone. Be sure your eyes do not skip as they go up the frame but follow as if drawing a line, as they did when following a finger. Soon you should have a good sense of motion. This is splendid for those unable to do the Long Swing, as it may even be done with a slight body sway while seated. However, in general, it should be done in addition to the Long Swing.

The Pencil Swing

As in all drills, practice makes for ease and perfection. The purpose of this drill is to reestablish the inner movement of the eye. Your eyes will feel easy, and you will have a sense of rhythm in your whole body. This drill may be done for any length of time and as many times a day as you desire. Your finger may be used as well as a pencil. Excellent for desk workers!

1) Hold a pencil about 8 inches in front of your eyes, the top level with your forehead as shown in figure 10. You may be seated, since this swing does not involve a body sway.

2) Swing your head in easy rhythm, humming a tune if you like. As your eyes pass the pencil, ignore it, looking beyond

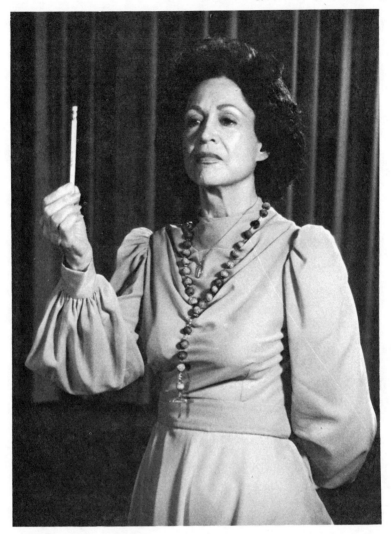

Figure 10. The Pencil Swing.

into the room. The pencil should soon seem to move in the opposite direction. If you do not have this illusion, it is because each time the eyes pass the pencil they look at it instead of beyond it.

The Dot-to-Dot Swing

Another good small movement exercise. Three steps are involved. First step:

1) Use a white card about 3 by 6 inches. Place a black dot in the center. The dot can be made from a piece of black paper or with pen and ink. Be sure it is black and about ¾ inch in diameter.

2) Place smaller black dots about ½ inch on either side of the center dot.

3) With a slight movement of your head, sweep your eyes from the outer left edge of the card across the dots to the right edge. In other words, from edge to edge, back and forth three or four times, with your nose following your eyes. By this time the dots should appear to be moving in the opposite direction.

4) Now close your eyes and repeat the swing several times. The appearance and movement of the dots may be more apparent than when your eyes are open. Open your eyes and repeat the drill.

Now move on to the second step:

1) With eyes open, look from the dot on the left side to the dot on the right, ignoring the center dot. This is a shorter shift and there will be less head movement. After a few times there will be a slight suggestion of a swing of the center dot. This swing will be more pronounced as you repeat it with your eyes closed, thinking the center dot as moving.

2) Repeat several times, eyes both opened and closed.

The "fine-tuning" is done in the final step:

1) The center dot is large enough to have definite sides. Shift your eyes from one side of it to the other. What does this

accomplish? It relaxes tension, and restores your eyes to the important 70-times-a-second shift previously mentioned.

2) It is good to follow two or three such open-eye swings with the eyes closed, performing the swing mentally. If you think of the dot swinging when your eyes are closed, it will be easier to sense the motion when you open your eyes again. If you learn to swing mentally, you can use this drill many times when circumstances prevent any other practice. It is excellent for releasing nerve tension. You cannot concentrate on this and think of anything else. It requires total attention. Remember: *the shorter the shift, the greater the relaxation.*

I once practiced this shift mentally while a dentist was drilling a tooth. He remarked, "You are not gripping the chair as most patients do." I was so absorbed in swinging the dot, I was hardly conscious of the drilling. Pain is always increased by tension, and if we can release tension by so simple an exercise, it is well worth learning.

As you sit in a room, "swing" a picture on the wall by looking first at the wall on one side and then on the other. You can swing a vase on a stand or one flower from a group in the vase, or perhaps the star atop a Christmas tree. So many things to put in motion. Learn to make a game of it.

OTHER DRILLS FROM OTHER SOURCES

In addition to the techniques taught by Dr. Bates, I have found other drills to be of equal value. While he lived, Dr. Bates taught many others who became teachers, and who expanded on his teachings throughout the world. I, too, have developed my own techniques based on Dr. Bates' work and have taught them at numerous yoga classes. I offer them to you in this section.

Juggling

One of the most relaxing methods and one that all students enjoy, regardless of age, is juggling balls.

Get two balls of a size that fits your hands nicely, brightly colored if possible. At first use only one ball. Toss it up with one hand and catch it with the other. Never allow your eyes to leave the ball. Watch it as it leaves one hand and you catch it with the other. To avoid stooping to retrieve missed balls, stand in front of a bed or chair. After a bit of practice you will always catch it. There is nothing more rewarding than this drill to give eye and mind coordination.

Next, take one ball in each hand. As you toss one up, still following it with your eyes, slip the ball from the other hand into the one the ball has just left. This juggling will soon become easy. If you hold one hand low, tossing the ball fairly high, it will give a good sweep to your eyes. You can also bounce the ball, following the same principle of eyes on the ball at all times.

In the training studio, the teacher and student sometimes play pitch ball together. At home you can do it with a member of your family. This is an excellent substitute for palming when it's hard to sit still very long. Learn to play ball with yourself and with others.

All of these drills can be done all day long as you adopt right seeing habits. You use your eyes constantly, so learn to use them correctly. For example, while you work around the house, learn to follow the movement of your hands. As you make a bed, follow the large swings and movements. As you peel a vegetable round and round, be aware of a short swing potential. Watch the iron swing back and forth, the hammer go up and down. Many times the hand works on its own, the eyes parked some place waiting your return. Let the hands and eyes join in the household tasks, resulting in excellent hand and mind coordination.

If you are an office worker, learn to follow the many movements of your hands with your eyes as you work. You will end your day less tired because your whole coordination has been better. In a nearby drawer keep the little dot card and a ball. Several times a day, when stress, tiredness, and tension develop, take a moment to swing the dot. Take the ball and toss it up, shifting from hand to hand. What a relief and release to tired eyes! Remember, one reason for tired eyes is that they fasten and stick on letters, print, or objects.

I remember a friend who, because she had lost the sight of one eye, was afraid to use the other. She was obsessed with "saving" her one eye. She cut herself off from all activity. She thought that by not using it she would somehow keep it "safe." Instead, her sight began to deteriorate. I directed her to these and the Bates drills and advised normal use of the eye. Her vision was restored. Not only that, but she became a different person as she once again resumed her active life. "Use it or lose it" is an adage familiar to all. It is certainly true with eyes. Your eyes were given for use. As windows of the soul, they should be used wisely and well.

Wall Chart Training

Using a wall chart to exercise the eyes is an excellent idea because it can be done frequently. Hang one over your desk while you work, for example; it's convenient because it's easy to look up from your work and exercise your eyes for a few minutes.

Prepare a chart similar to the kind found in an eye doctor's office. Figure 11 on page 72 shows one example. The chart you make should be at least 8½ by 11 inches. Choose either letters of the alphabet or numbers. Follow the format shown in the figure—the top line should be the largest, the next line a little smaller, and so on down to the bottom of the chart. The lines should be an equal distance apart, and each letter should be an equal distance from the others. Sit 5 to 15 feet away. Begin at the upper left-hand corner of the chart, focus your eyes clearly on the letter there, then move to the next, following the figures across the chart to the right. Then bring your eyes back to the second line, on the left, and

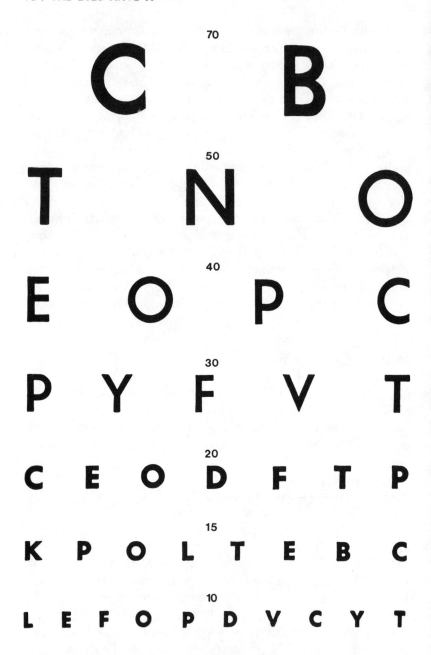

Figure 11. A wall chart for exercising the eyes.

repeat. Thus, you will be scanning every letter from left to right, beginning at the largest and proceeding to the smallest.

As your eyes fall on each letter, make a circle (or a square) with your eyes around that letter before proceeding to the next. Do this exercise twice a day if possible. Then remove the top line and raise all the lines upward, and add an even smaller line to the bottom. Repeat the exercises for another week and then reduce the letters again. Follow this procedure until it is difficult for you to see the letters on the last line. Train your eyes to focus on the small figures again and again, bringing them clearly into view. You will find that they suddenly become clearer and clearer until you are reading them easily at a distance. Blink often.

Remove that chart completely. Find an old book with large type that you do not mind destroying. Remove the pages. One by one place them on the wall and sit back far enough so that it is difficult to read the writing. Train your eyes to do so. Do not practice too long at a session. Blink often. From 2 to 5 minutes is sufficient in the beginning.

The Cross-Eyed Drill

Focus on your finger held at arm's length. Bring your finger to the tip of your nose, following it with your eyes. You will be looking "cross-eyed." Repeat the procedure several times, then rest your eyes. Later practice this near-far shifting without your finger.

The Pinhole Pursuit

Purchase pinhole spectacles—glasses with dark lenses containing many pinholes (available at most health stores). Remove your glasses (if you wear them) and wear the pinhole glasses as long as possible during each day. Take them off for resting your eyes, but wear them again and again during the course of the day. Try watching television with them. Looking at the world through the pinholes is one of the most marvelous eye exercises possible. You will find that you are able to read the finest print while reading through the pinholes. Repeated use of these pinhole spectacles could, sooner or later, allow you to discard your glasses.

Variation on the Long Swing

Adopt a Long Swing movement of the body from side to side with your hands extended in front of you (see figure 12).

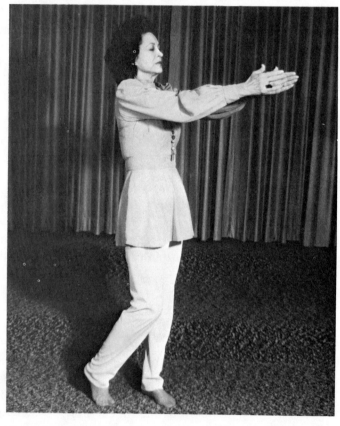

Figure 12. A variation on the Long Swing, where you focus your attention on the space between your two palms. Stance is the same as shown in figure 9 on page 64.

Keep your attention focused on the space between your two palms as you swing your hands in a wide expanse from side to side. Keep your shoulders parallel with the walls. Begin with fifty complete swings and increase to one hundred.

Mental Image Drills

While lying in bed or sitting in a chair, whichever is most relaxing, close your eyes and picture your nose as a long, soft pencil. Before you is a sheet of white paper. On this paper, with your long soft pencil, draw a large circle. Keep it perfectly round. Note that your head swings in a circular direction, down and over and above and down. Do this several times from right to left, then reverse from left to right. Repetition makes the line very black against the white paper. Think of it as the rim of a wheel.

A wheel must have spokes. Draw a line from the lower rim to the upper rim. Repeat several times until the line is very black. Be sure your head is in an easy, rhythmical swing—chin down, chin up—closed eyes following the mental picture of lines being drawn.

Next, without dipping your chin, draw a line from shoulder to shoulder, from the left side of the rim to the right side, crossing the center line. Then reverse. Repeat a few times.

Now draw a spoke from the lower left to the upper right, swinging your head in a diagonal motion. Repeat several times. Then, draw a spoke in the opposite direction, from the lower right to the upper left.

Now that the spokes are in the wheel, it must have a hubcap. With a forward thrust of your chin, place a dot at the very center of your hubcap. You have completed your optical wheel.

Close your eyes. For sake of variety, mentally take a fresh sheet of paper. With the same long nose pencil, start at the lower left corner of the paper and draw a line to the upper right. Make a loop across to the upper left, then diagonally across to the lower right. Add a loop at the bottom to the lower left. You have drawn a large figure 8. Go over this several times and reverse the direction. On another sheet of paper, draw a figure 8 crosswise, horizontally on the paper.

You will think of other things to draw with your nose pencil, such as special words, your name, the names of cities, and so on. You can sometimes do this as sky writing. You have seen words written across the sky with trails of vapor from an airplane. Picture your nose drawing words across the sky and, with a big breath, watch them disappear. These mental drills are especially good to stimulate the imagination as well as to ease tense and stiff neck and shoulder muscles, which, by the way, may be caused by tense eyes. Vivid imagination and clear mental pictures are major aids in maintaining health for the eyes.

Correct breathing is imperative for healthy eyes. Tight, stiff eyes often develop in people who forget to breathe when they are making an effort to see. Good vision is dependent on good circulation, and correct breathing stimulates circulation. Do establish proper breathing habits. Occasionally take a deep breath. If you exhale a deep breath quickly, it will project a fresh blood supply up into the eyes.

Often take a little quick breath, exhaling with a sigh, as a sleepy puppy does when he lies down to rest. Picture the relaxation of animals. What is more relaxed than a cat in front of a fire? Try to emulate this in your relaxation. Establish these health habits for your eyes and reap the reward of excellent vision.

Making Photographs Come Alive

Select a picture in a newspaper or book. Close one eye. With the open eye, imagine you are seeing the head of a pin in the center of the picture. Suddenly the picture will assume three dimensions. It will actually seem to come to life. Practicing this illusion improves visual depth perception, enabling you to see different objects in their true positions relative to each other.

Strengthening Muscular Control

Hold one end of a string against the end of your nose. Stretch the string straight out before you about 36 inches and attach the other end to a window frame or nail. At first you will see only one string, but continue looking at the far end of the string and suddenly you will see two strings.

As long as you are actually seeing with both eyes, you will see the two strings coming to a *V* point, regardless of where you look along the one string. At the *V* point, the two strings appear to cross, forming an X. By closing either eye, you will find that the illusory string you thought you were seeing with your left eye is actually seen by the right eye, and vice versa. Place your fingers on a point closer to the nose. See the two strings.

See how close to your nose you can move your fingers along the string and still see two strings—optimally 3 or 4 inches. You will be tempted to close one eye, but that defeats the purpose of the drill. Continued daily practice strengthens eye muscles and rests the eyes. It will also delay the need for reading glasses.

FOR THE SENIOR CITIZEN

Seniors with failing sight often give up in despair. In the words of Dr. J.H. Tilden, a Denver physician who became a naturopath: "The diseases of old age are not due to old age. They are due to wrong life." If cataracts have been diagnosed, some people are apt to sit for hours staring into space, unhappy and worried. Interest in and practice of easy Bates drills gives them a new goal. The worry of waiting for possible blindness can be totally negated as eyesight begins to respond. The results, in both better eyesight and a happier outlook, can be amazing. Palming is an easy exercise for the elderly, and if they can listen to music or a good taperecorded lecture, so much the better, for it will help encourage mental pictures. It also may be a good time for someone to read something to them, but the subject must be of interest. An article from *Reader's Digest,* perhaps, or from *Science Digest.* Or *Christian Science.* Or *Science of Mind.* Or *Unity* literature. Or a degree lesson from Astara.

Sunning should be done at first with their backs toward the sun and spanning the bright sky with their swings. Some may find the light difficult at first. They may be taught a gentle swing while sitting in a chair. Have them hold an arm of the chair with each hand to steady themselves while they sway gently from side to side, keeping their eyes in the same position as for the Long Swing. Get them interested in gardening, but be sure it is performed before 10:00 A.M. or after 4:00 P.M. While you want to be sure they avoid glare, do not condemn them to a darkened room! The light may bother them at first, but with perseverance they will quickly overcome it.

In a car, have them keep their eyes moving from one side of the street to the other. Warn them not to stare straight ahead. Often the motion of the car will enable them to read large print on the billboards, because the motion prevents staring at the words and they see them more as a flash vision. You can assist by asking, "What does this next billboard advertise?" Get them interested in *seeing*. How much they can see once they attain muscle relaxation will amaze you and them. Get them a large ball and have them toss it from one hand to the other. A paddle with the ball attached by a rubber band is good for them to use.

Part 3

YOGA AND THE EYES

.

One must make a daily practice of wrong living to remain ill, for nature is constantly at work throwing off disease.

—Dr. J.H. Tilden

Yogic Exercises to Strengthen Eyes

It is well recognized that the muscles of the body should be exercised to remain healthy. Otherwise they become saturated with wastes and toxins. Why should it be any different with the eyes? They are surrounded by muscles that should be exercised. If they are not, stagnation and toxins congest them just as with other muscles; and the debris flows into and through the eyes, finally resulting in deterioration.

To *maintain* healthy eyes, they must be exposed to *light*. They must be fed with certain enzymes from the proper foods, and they must be exercised and stimulated. These things are also required to *regain* healthy eyes. The eyes can recover perfect health just as other parts of the body can. Why should the eye be different, unless some degenerative disease is present? However, the eye itself is *rarely* the original seat of a degenerative disease; it is usually a victim.

As long as eye muscles are kept resilient, relaxed, and balanced, as long as the diet contains natural foods, as long as the eye is occasionally stimulated through inflowing light rays, the function of seeing—which is the true purpose of the eye—should remain unimpaired. Neglect of any of the above results in eye strain, tension, poor circulation, defective lens, pressure, toxic buildup.

At one time it was believed that once the shape of the eye was altered, resulting in nearsightedness, farsightedness, or astigmatism, such a refractive error became permanent. But both the Bates System of correction and the yogic techniques taught and practiced by renowned yogis have proved such a belief to be false. Both systems explain that the damage results from unequal tension of the six muscles that attach to the outer tissues of the eyeball.

Throughout the previous section, I have written with dedication about the Bates method of eyesight improvement. But I am also a yogi and have practiced yoga for many years, including methods for improving the eyesight. I shall present yogic techniques for eye improvement, and then you may decide your personal preference.

The Clock Technique

The following is the famous clock technique. It may be practiced standing, sitting, or lying down. I usually practice it lying down, before I rise in the morning, along with other isometric exercises, which I presented in *The Book of Beginning Again.*[2] One morning I practice the stretching, tensing, and relaxing exercises lying flat on my back; the next morning, lying on my right side; on the third, lying on my left side. The next day, I return to those done lying on the back and continue my rotation. But faithfully, every morning, I practice one special exercise lying on my back—the clock technique. It is for the eyes. Figure 13 shows an example of this exercise. Here is the technique, which is practiced from a supine position:

1) Lie on your back (or sit or stand), squeeze your eyes tightly, open them and blink—light, fluttering blinks. Repeat three times. As you do this, strike light blows on your temples with the heel of each hand. Now take a deep breath, hold it, then release it in a long sigh. You have just opened the arteries and started a flow of fresh blood into the entire eye area, bringing oxygen and life force into restricted muscles, stimulating circulation.

2) Now imagine the face of a huge clock suspended on the ceiling. First, focus your eyes on the center of the clock face, directly above you. Now raise your eyes upward as far as

[2]Earlyne Chaney, *The Book of Beginning Again, or, A Funny Thing Happened on My Way to Heaven,* (Upland, CA: Astara, 1981).

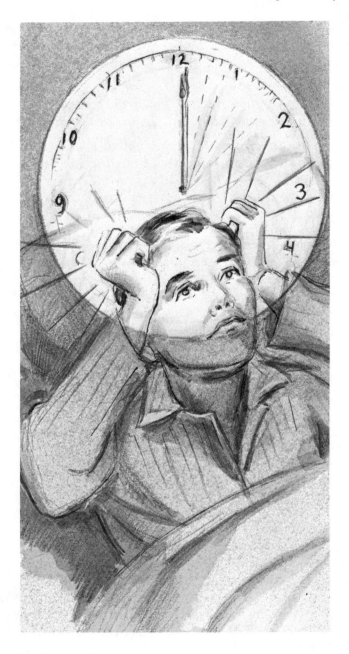

Figure 13. The Clock Technique.

possible toward twelve o'clock, still striking your temples. Return your eyes to the center of the clock, then lower them to six o'clock, as far as possible. Return to the center.

3) Turn your eyes to the right, to three o'clock, still striking your temples. Return them again to the center. Now turn them as far as possible to the left, to nine o'clock, then center.

4) Now raise them upward to one o'clock and then back to the center. Then downward to seven o'clock and back to the center, toward ten o'clock and back to the center, toward four o'clock and back to the center. Repeat this procedure several times, continuing to strike light blows.

It is extremely important that you bring your eyes back to the center of the clock each time, pausing a brief second to rest them. After repeating the procedure several times, turn your eyes downward to six o'clock and make a large circle around the clock clockwise with both eyes, pause, and then counterclockwise. Rest your eyes a moment with your palms covering them. Continue palming until your eyes have returned to total relaxation.

The percussion blows on the temples have a wonderfully invigorating effect on your eyes and will surely aid in improving your vision. Great care should be taken not to overdo these exercises the first few times. Move gently, to avoid straining any unused muscles.

The Neck Stretch

Now perform the following neck exercise (see figure 14). Sitting upright, drop your head down, stretching your neck. Lift your chin toward the ceiling, stretching your throat. Now try to touch your left ear to your left shoulder, stretching; then your right ear to your right shoulder, stretching. Now turn your head as far to the right as possible, looking over your right shoulder; then to the left.

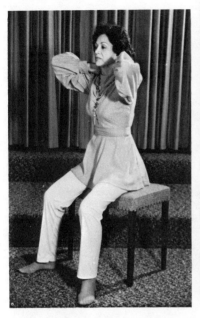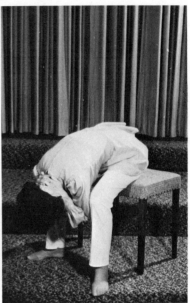

Figure 14. The Neck Stretch.

Drop your head forward as far as possible, then slowly rotate your head to your left shoulder. Slowly let it fall backward. Rotate it next to the right, and drop it forward again. Pause for a moment of relaxation, then reverse the rotation. Repeat the rotation each way several times, very slowly.

Now place your hands on the back of your head, near the nape of your neck, fingers interlocked. With your knees apart, take a deep breath. As you bend forward to lower your head between your knees, expel your breath vigorously. With the interlocked fingers, press and pump your head downward as far as possible, stretching your neck.

These exercises not only improve eyesight, they align your head with your spine and release the flow of ingathered toxins so that your entire body is benefited.

Recharging the Optic Nerve

Secure a gold, copper, or silver coin and place it about 12 inches in front of your feet on the floor as shown in figure 15. Gold is preferable because it is the most magnetic. Copper is the second choice because it is more magnetic than silver.

Bend forward, keeping your spine and neck in line, elbows on knees. If it is necessary to focus your eyes, hold them wide open with the tips of your forefingers and thumbs; close the other fingers. Gaze at the coin a few

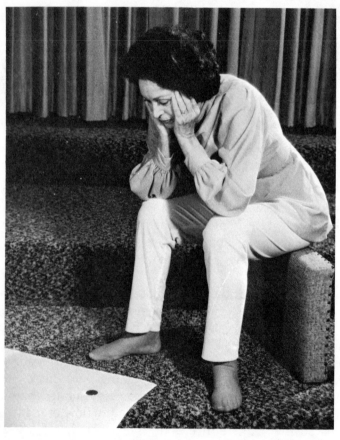

Figure 15. Recharging the optic nerve by focusing on a small object—in this case a penny.

minutes, still holding your eyes open. Now revolve your eyes around the coin in circles, from left to right, just as you did with the imagined clock face. Gradually enlarge the circle. On your final rotation, pause on each of the clock numerals. Now reverse your rotation from right to left.

Then, still leaning forward, rest your chin on your palms and gaze at the coin. Tears should form. Close your eyes and relax them completely. Palm a moment. Rub your eyes with a slight pressure, taking care not to hurt them. Open your eyes again, only partially, and gaze at the coin a few moments. During this exercise always keep your body bent forward with elbows on knees.

As you gaze with half-closed eyes at the coin, mentally try to move it—up and down, right and left. Then attempt to pick it up mentally. Contract the muscles of the eyes and forehead if necessary. Make a true attempt to move the coin with your eyes. Finish the exercise by closing your eyes and palming, resting and relaxing for a few moments.

Recharging with Blue Light

Secure a 200-watt blue electric light bulb, or as near this strength as possible. Using an extension cord or a cord from the ceiling, see that it is placed about 3 feet in front of you, aligned with your eyes.

Sit with spine erect, chin in, head up. Gaze into the blue light with eyes partially closed for approximately 1 minute. Then close your eyes. Concentrate on the afterimage of the blue light. See the face of the clock mentally before you, in the center of the blue light.

With your eyes still closed, lift them to twelve o'clock, the point between your eyebrows. Return to the center of the clock and open your eyes, gazing for a moment into the blue light. Close your eyes again, see the afterimage, then turn them to three o'clock. Return to the center, open your eyes, and gaze at the blue light. Close them, see the afterimage, then look downward to six o'clock, then back to the center. Continue this, completing the face of the clock, each time opening your eyes to see the blue light again, then superimposing a number on the afterimage all the way around the face of the clock.

The idea is to see the afterimage of the blue light with the number you have chosen superimposed on it. This exercise is invaluable for restoring eyesight, as well as for developing clairvoyance.

Sun Afterimage

This is similar to the previous exercise, except that instead of the blue light you will be using the sun. This exercise should be practiced only before 10:00 A.M. or after 4:00 P.M. because it is not advisable to look into the sun at any other time.

Sit erect facing the sun. Look briefly into the sun, then close your eyes, and raise them to the twelve o'clock position. Hold this image before you as long as possible, gazing hard at the afterimage of the sun with the number 12 superimposed on it. Keep your eyes upturned to the spot between your eyebrows.

When the image fades, open your eyes again to look briefly into the sun. Close them, and turn your eyes to three o'clock. Hold the afterimage there until it fades away. Each time the image begins to move away from the far right, draw it back, slowly allowing it to return to the center, straight ahead. When the afterimage fades, open your eyes to gaze at the sun again. Repeat this at the six o'clock and nine o'clock positions until you have covered the entire face of your clock. Each time, open your eyes briefly to see the sun, closing them to see the afterimage with the numeral of the clock superimposed on it. This exercise may also be practiced during a full moon.

If your eyes are supersensitive to the sun, it may be advisable to wear a green shade for a few weeks—the kind often worn by tennis players or golfers—so that your eyes are not exposed to the direct sunlight.

Word Images

Secure a sheet of paper with writing on it, either typewritten or handwritten. It may be a section of newspaper print or a page torn from an old book or magazine. Make sure you are unable to read the print without your glasses. Select one word on the page and paste something over all the rest of the copy.

Sit bending forward with your neck and spine in line, elbows on knees. Let your neck crouch into the shoulders if you feel more comfortable. Hold the sheet you have prepared between the forefinger and thumb of each hand.

Close your eyes tightly with your forehead contracted. Open your eyes and blink rapidly. Gaze at the one word on the paper for about 1 minute. Blink often. The word will sometimes fade completely away, then return clearly. Gaze at the word until you can hold it clearly in your vision. Palm and rest the eyes. Practice this exercise often. You may practice as long as 2 hours at a time, though only a few minutes will perform wonders.

As you continue practicing, cover everything on the page except two words, then three words, then an entire line, then a complete paragraph. Follow the instructions above, gazing easily at the copy until you are able to read it clearly. Do not strain. Blink often. Be sure to read the same copy over and over again until you have mastered seeing it clearly before you change the copy.

Do not neglect to rotate your eyes during the day, with your eyes closed. Occasionally open them wide, gazing steadily ahead without blinking for a moment.

DR. SOM'S HEALING TECHNIQUES

Mystics usually employ the use of the crystal ball only as a means to develop clairvoyance, but Dr. Som used it to cure and heal the physical eyes. He placed the crystal ball 7 or 8 inches from the eyes at eye level. The patient was asked to gaze wide-eyed at the crystal ball until the tears came, while breathing audibly and deeply. With the appearance of tears, the eyes were closed and the breath became quiet and gentle.

The closed eyes/quiet breathing session was continued for about 2 minutes; then the exercise was repeated. The gazing, tears, audible and quiet breathing all contribute considerably to the health of the eyes—and the development of the Third Eye of clairvoyance.

Dr. Som also encouraged rolling the eyes, not only for better vision but because the exercise also stimulated the inner organs. He prepared a circular chart with the numbers 1, 2, 3, 4 on it, clockwise. The instructions were to face the chart and roll the eyes from left to right, clockwise. Rolling the eyes was performed simultaneously with rolling the tongue around the teeth in the same direction and inhaling at the same time.

With the completion of the circle, the eyes were rolled counterclockwise, with the tongue following the same movement while the breath was exhaled. There were nine inhalations and nine exhalations. Then a brief meditation followed, with the eyes closed and quiet, slow breathing, palming if possible.

Dr. Som's Cross Eyes

Sit quietly, spine erect, with your eyes open. Imagine a clock before your eyes. Lift your eyes upward to twelve o'clock, then to the center. Now turn your eyes to focus on the tip of your nose so that they are crossed. Now turn the eyes to three o'clock, then to the center, and cross eyes at the nose tip; then six o'clock, and so on, all around the clock face. Reverse and roll your eyes completely around the clock; then reverse them the other way.

This can be done anytime, anywhere—waiting for a bus, waiting for an elevator, sitting at your desk, lying on a slantboard, taking a walk. For the center, focus on any object directly on a level with your eyes. Palm afterward if possible.

This particular exercise is one of my favorites. It is of utmost benefit. Focusing on your nose tip also stimulates development of the Third Eye for clairvoyance, and the simultaneous development of the right brain—the brain of intuition.

Walking with the Eyes

Are you taking a daily walk? If not, try your best to form such a habit. Walk at least around your block—a mile would be even better. As you walk, forget your problems and turn your attention to mental alertness. Concentrate on increasing your powers of perception, observing everything that is happening around you.

Focus your eyes fully, first on one thing and then another. Select first an object near at hand, then immediately an object in the far distance, so that your eyes are continuously adjusting their vision—accommodating, shifting. Look at something on one side of the street and then the other; something down on the ground, then something high in the air. Concentrate on moving your eyes and your head simultaneously.

The Blue Light Exercise

This exercise should be practiced just before retiring. Purchase an 8-watt blue electric light bulb. Connect it to an extension cord or lamp. Sit on a low stool or firm pillow so that your elbows rest on your upraised knees. Place the blue blub on a level with your eyes. Sit about 3 feet from it. Gaze steadily at the blue light for about 2 minutes or until the tears form. Go immediately to bed without washing the tears away. This also can be done using the light of a candle in a darkened room. Practice this exercise every other night. Gradually increase to 5 minutes. Let the tears flow freely.

In the morning, bathe your eyes in salt water solution in a glass eye cup. Use ½ teaspoon of sea salt to 1 cup of warm distilled water.

The Concentration Chart

On the center of a white sheet of paper, paste or draw a black dot. Sit at a table and place this concentration chart 4 feet away from you. Gaze at the dot in the center without blinking your eyes. Keep your eyes half closed. Then drop your head as if attempting to touch your right shoulder with your ear, but keep your eyes focused on the black dot.

Now tilt your head backward as far as possible, with your eyes focused on the dot. Now drop your head as far to the left as possible, then drop your head down on your chest. Turn and tilt your face in all directions, keeping focused on the dot.

Self-Massage

Tension and rigidity of the muscles of the neck also cause impaired eyesight, for blood circulation is cut off from the arteries of the head, which are buried deep in the neck. However, blood returns from the head through veins that pass through the tissues of the neck near the surface. Therefore, when the muscles of the neck become tensed, they press against the veins, causing the blood to be closed off inside the head. The brain cells suffer, and so do the eyes, being denied their supply of renewed life force. Actually, the entire body is affected by this congestion in the brain. It commonly results in headaches.

Headaches, of course, can be controlled by pain pills and caused to disappear, but the damage to the eyes is not so obvious. We are only aware of the need for stronger glasses —or an operation for cataracts or glaucoma.

The exercise of rotating your head on your neck overcomes a great deal of this tension. The following exercise also is for relaxing the neck muscles so that the blood flows easily into and out of the brain, charging the brain cells and the eyes with renewed life force.

Place the fingers of your left hand on the bones of your neck, the tips pointed toward the bones, the hand arched, as shown in figure 16 on page 94. Place the fingers of your other hand in the same position, backing them against the fingers of your left hand. Grasp the muscles of your neck in your hands, and pull outward as if you were pulling the muscles away from bones. Alternate pulling with your hands. Pull on the muscles on the sides of the neck, then directly over the spinal cord. Pull and relax...pull and relax.

Then grasp the flesh firmly and rotate your head— downward, upward, backward, from side to side. If you suffer from tension headaches, this technique often releases the tension.

It is also a good idea every now and then to lie on a slant, with your feet higher than your head. Relax every muscle, including your neck muscles, so that the blood can flow into your brain and out again, rejuvenating brain cells, muscles, and tissues of the eyes. If possible, spend at least 10 minutes a day "slanting." Perform the clock, the cross-eyes, or any of the other exercises you wish. Palm if you can spare the time.

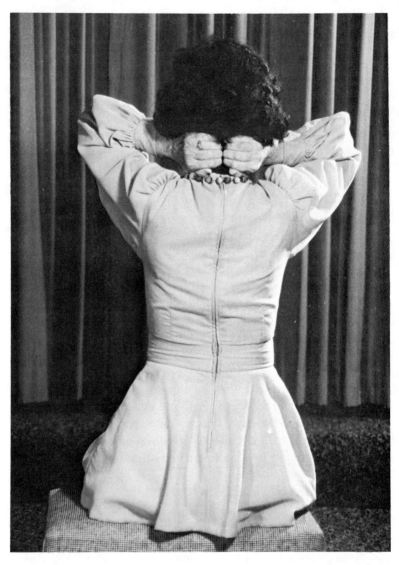

Figure 16. Massaging the muscles at the base of the skull. Many of us experience tension in this area, and this tension can lead to impaired vision.

Training the Side Vision

When riding in a car—but not while driving!—lift your hands to block the vision straight before you and force yourself to see passing objects—houses, trees, telephone poles, wires—from the corner of your eyes. This helps train the side "muscles" of the eyeballs.

Strengthening the Brain Center

Sit in the dark, with only the blue light bulb—either the strong or the weak wattage. Gaze directly at the light. Drop your chin onto your chest, with your eyes still focused on the blue light. Tilt your chin backward, still holding your gaze. Turn your head in every direction, keeping the light always in your range of vision—down and back, to every side, to the right and to the left. Rotate your head around and around on your neck from left to right and right to left, always keeping your gaze on the blue light. This exercise stimulates the muscles around your eyes and the fibers of the eye itself.

Now turn off the blue light, sit erect in the dark, feet flat on the floor, hands in your lap. Drop your chin onto your chest, and inhale a complete yogic breath through the nostrils. While exhaling slowly through your nostrils, pull your navel in and up. At the same time raise your head and sit very erect. Continue breathing through your nostrils.

Now, with eyes open, see the image of your clock face before you. Rotate your eyes around the clock, and reverse, as usual. Tilt your head backward and gaze directly at the ceiling. Keep your eyes from blinking for as long as possible. Breathe long, deep breaths. Now repeat the exercise of rolling your eyes clockwise and counterclockwise. Then close them and rest.

ACUPRESSURE TECHNIQUES

There are millions of Chinese—but few wear glasses! Dr. Som studied acupressure from several experts, including a skilled Chinese acupuncturist. This Chinese master told him that the Chinese attributed their good eyes to the practice of a few special eye exercises, based on the science of acupuncture, requiring only 10 minutes. These four simple techniques should be practiced twice a day.

While sitting, meditate on some happy place or time and begin massaging key pressure points located around the eyes. These points are shown in figure 17 and further described below. Massaging these points apparently relaxes the focusing muscles, releases tension, and stimulates blood circulation. The hands should be clean, and the massage should be firm but without excessive pressure. Each exercise should be repeated at least eight times, preferably twelve times.

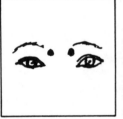

A) With your elbows on a table, place your thumbs just inside the eyebrow corners near the root of your nose. Let your fingers curl on your forehead. Massage lightly and slowly, four times in one direction, then reverse.

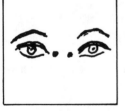

B) Place the thumb and index fingers of one hand on each side of the nose bridge at the corner of each eye. Press upward, then downward, slowly and lightly but firmly.

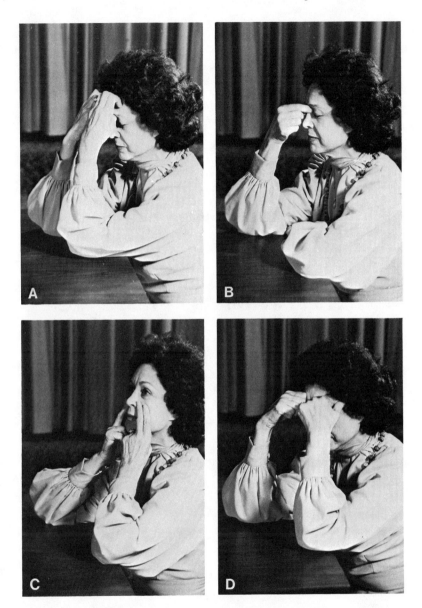

Figure 17. Acupressure points for relaxing the eyes and relieving tension. The points shown here are a) root of nose, b) bridge of nose, c) jawbone, and d) temple.

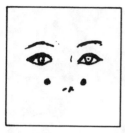

C) Place your thumbs on your jaws. Place your index and middle fingers against both sides of your nose. Lower your middle finger, leaving your index finger on a strategic pressure point. Massage firmly and slowly.

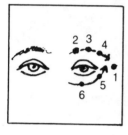

D) Place your thumbs on your temples. Curl your fingers under. Using the side of your index finger, rub outward on the pressure points, following the chart: 1-2-3-4-5-6. Keep your thumbs on your temples, using your index finger to apply the pressure and perform the rubbing.

Since Dr. Som taught me this important eye exercise, I have seen it extolled in various media. Dr. Som firmly believed that, if this exercise were started early enough, one would never need glasses, and glasses could be discarded by most. Dr. Som never owned a pair of glasses. He lived almost one hundred years and was still performing chiropractic adjustments until the day of his death. He was a strict vegetarian. He used a magnifying glass only for reading very fine print.

Part 4

Beware and Be Aware: Prevention and Cure

After securing a normal body and mind, then the mind must be trained toward right thinking by being fed units of truth.

—Dr. J.H. Tilden

Do's and Don'ts for Healthy Eyes

For healthy eyes, there are many do's and don'ts. I'd rather say there are things about which you should be aware in order to beware.

Ultraviolet light: Ultraviolet rays can be dangerous. That is why those who lie directly exposed to the downpouring rays of midday sunlight—with or without dark glasses—are extremely foolish. They invite cataracts. Dark glasses are penetrated by these rays, so they offer little protection. But they *should* be worn if you insist on such sunbathing.

Never suntan under an ultraviolet lamp, either in the home or in a suntan parlor. They are dangerous. Even dark glasses will not offer total protection to the eyes. The rays can penetrate the glass and your closed eyelids. The glasses may even accentuate the heat on your eyeballs. These rays could cause cataracts. Sunlamp rays (ultraviolet) are certainly the cause of premature aging of the skin, just like sun rays at high noon. They greatly increase the risk of skin cancer. Remember that electric log fireplaces often emit harmful ultraviolet rays, especially if there is a red glowing element. One should never gaze into such artificial rays.

Electric light bulbs simultaneously emit infrared, white light, and ultraviolet rays. The glass container offers some protection for the eyes. Plain glass bulbs should not be used unless they are so screened as to prevent looking directly at the white-hot filament. The best bulbs for home or office are made of opal glass, which completely shields the eyes from the damaging filament.

Fluorescent lighting: Cool-white fluorescent lighting—used extensively in schools, offices, factories, and now even in homes—is harmful not only to the eyes but also to your teeth and all of your bones. It also drains your energy. The light makes it difficult for the body to absorb calcium, and when calcium is leached from the body, the eyes, teeth, and bones certainly suffer.

Fluorescent lights that produce light similar to that of the sun are now available but at a considerably higher price than the cool-white. But safety for your eyes makes such a choice imperative. Recent research indicates skin cancer could result from exposure to cool-white fluorescent tubes. Never work or live under cool-white fluorescents. Make sure they are "full spectrum" tubes. There is a brand called Vita-Lite Full Spectrum fluorescent tubes and also a brand called Kiva Lights. Ask at your local hardware store.

Television and eyes: It should be remembered that the picture tube in a television set is radioactive. Thus, exposure at close range can be extremely detrimental to the eyes. It is universally known that one should stay at least 6 feet from black-and-white sets and 12 feet from color television. Exposure to television radiation may be the cause of many unknown and unrecognized illnesses, especially eye ailments. Unfortunately, only time will be able to tell the long-range effects of radiation on the eyes. The screen should be about eye level. A light should be left on in the room. During commercials, palm to relieve any tension and to rest the eyes.

Eyedrops: Prescription and over-the-counter drops usually contain drugs that, when absorbed into the body, are toxic to the system, especially for the young and the elderly. Some contain only borax and salt—which cost only pennies to produce yet are sold at exorbitant prices. If you want to duplicate these solutions, add 1 part of boric acid to 25 parts of distilled water.

Over the counter drugs that "get the red out" can be dangerous. They usually contain benzalkonium chloride, tetrahydrozoline hydrochloride, and antipyrine. These drops constrict or dilate the blood vessels, which in itself is an unwise practice. It is the *cause* of redness that should be corrected. Constricting the flow of blood into the eye prevents the very flow of life force needed. Avoid using them. Turn to the natural remedies suggested here and by other naturalists. See a holistic ophthalmologist if the red persists. The red may be a warning of something needing attention.

Good eyewashes, from natural sources, are now available at health stores. They are totally different from the drugstore products and may be used with confidence. But if eyes are red, they may need more than an eyewash. They may need herbal treatments. If redness persists, see a doctor.

Tight collars: Never wear tight collars. Worn habitually, they cut off circulation. To aid circulation, make a daily habit of splashing the face, especially the eyes, with alternate hot and cold water, ending with cold.

Baby bathing: Care should be taken when bathing a baby near any kind of artificial heat, whether coal fire, oil heater, electric or gas fire. Mothers who wear glasses should be aware that their eyes are protected from the heat of the fire, whereas the eyes of the infant are not. Such heat could damage baby eyes and even the exposed naked skin.

Don't rub the eyes: Some people habitually rub their eyes, which in itself is a sure indication of a need for release from tension. Rubbing is not the answer. Never rub; palm instead. *Rubbing is especially injurious during a fever.* It causes visual disturbances. Myopia (nearsightedness) may occur because the white part of the eye is stretched out of shape by repeated rubbing. When this distortion happens, the image focuses in front of the retina, like a camera out of focus. As a result, you can see near (nearsightedness) but not far unless you wear corrective eye glasses.

Never rub your eye when there's a speck in it. The dirt or foreign object could scratch the cornea. Lift the upper eyelid over the lower lid, which will stimulate tears. Let the tears wash out the object. Or blow the nostril opposite to the afflicted eye. This will sometimes help remove the offending object.

Don't squint!: Most people, when viewing a distant object, tend to squint. Or they squint when walking on a sunny day. Don't! You are damaging the ciliary muscles of your eyes—the muscles that encircle the lens of the eye. The tug of squinting shortens the eyeball to bring objects into better focus on your retina, the membrane lining the back of the eye. But constant squinting weakens the ciliary muscles—just as constantly stretching a rubber band will eventually cause it to lose its elasticity.

Before looking at a distant object or before squinting in bright sunlight, blink rapidly several times. Then squeeze your eyes and open them widely—bulge them—a few times. This will stimulate the ciliary muscles so that the distant object becomes clear.

Microwave ovens: Microwave ovens are constantly suspected of being associated with the formation of cataracts because of leaking radiation. This is a controversial issue, however. Those opposed to this proposition have an equally substantial argument that the ovens are tested and safe.

Do wear protective goggles: When performing a do-it-yourself job around the house, wear protective goggles. Recently a friend decided to mow his own lawn. The motor struck a pile of debris, sending a particle to lodge in his eye, which became red, swollen, and painful. He inserted a couple of chia seeds, knowing their sticky substance could pick up any object and eject it. No object came out. Then he bathed his eye with eyebright herb tea several times a day for ten days, until it returned to normal.

But donning goggles would have been advisable. Many accidents causing blindness occur around the house—breaking glass, metal chips from grinders, wood chips from power saws, and flying objects from lawn mowers. Do protect your eyes with goggles when performing hazardous activities, even at home.

Cosmetic dangers: Old cosmetics should be discarded. They become contaminated—especially mascara—and have caused innumerable eye infections and some cases of blindness. Mascara should never be kept longer than three months because of a buildup of dangerous bacteria and fungus that, applied to an eye with only a slight blemish or scratch, could cause serious infection. If a mascara brush loaded with contaminated mascara should scratch the cornea (the clear, domed membrane covering the front of the eyeball), serious problems could result.

Bags under your eyes: Try a cucumber pack. Peel a cucumber and crush it. Add the white of an egg and an ounce of witch hazel to the cucumber. Mix and wrap in an oblong piece of cloth, preferably cheesecloth. Place the pack in the freezer until firm. Lie down, place the pack across your eyes, and relax for 10 minutes. The bags will be aided—and also your crow's feet and eyesight.

Stir a heaping teaspoon of yeast flakes into a bowl of milk until dissolved. Add an ice cube. Saturate two pure cotton pads in the milk, lie with your head on a large towel, and cover your eyes with the pads. The milk reduces bags under eyes; the yeast cells destroy wrinkles.

Dip a mint, sage, or camomile tea bag into a cup of ice water. Apply to eyes and relax.

Eye creams: Avoid eye creams that are heavy in texture and contain artificial coloring and perfume. An oil or cream too heavy will not absorb easily and could cause drooping in the muscles around the eye. Vitamin E oil is excellent if not too heavy. If heavy, mix it with aloe vera gel. Added coloring and fragrance can be dangerous to eye tissue, irritating and inflaming.

Do remember the miraculous Fanie eye cream, containing niacin, mentioned earlier. It is light and greaseless, vanishing almost immediately into the skin. Fanie Products also makes a fantastic face mask that not only tightens skin and removes wrinkles but, patted near and on the eyes, firms up loose skin over the eyelids—thus aiding eyesight. Order from Dr. Valjean McGinty, whose address is given in the appendix.

Lampshades and eyes: Colored lampshades should be chosen with care—and with an awareness of color and its effect. A red lampshade, while admittedly creating a sense of cozy warmth, could be very irritating to eyes. Overstimulation creates tired eyes. Pink shades, on the other hand, are excellent. Yellow offers mild stimulation to both eyes and mind. Green shades, offering an opposite effect to red, are cold and mildly sedative. Blue can be cool and restful. Beige with almost any color is excellent.

Proper lighting: Those who habitually read in bed should have light coming from behind and above their heads. You should read in a comfortable reclining, half-sitting position. Never lie on one side, resting on an elbow, while reading by the light of a bedside pedestal. Such an unnatural posture imposes a serious strain on the external eye muscles, resulting in defective vision.

Many bedrooms have a single light suspended from the middle of the ceiling. Reading from such a source is unwise. The light is in front of the eyes and beats down on them. For reading, close work, or desk work, the light source should always be behind and above the head, falling directly on the reading material.

A bathroom should always be brightly lighted. The light switch should never be within reach of one immersed in water, either in bath or shower. Touching it could result in electrocution.

Rotating the eye: Keep a teakettle of boiled water on your stove. When your eyes feel tired, fill a glass eyecup with this purified water, add a pinch of salt, and while the solution is applied to the eye, perform the clock face rotation exercise.

Squeezing: Pause several times a day and squeeze your eyes shut, then relax them. This stimulates the blood of the entire optic area. If you inhale and hold your breath while squeezing, then relax with a vigorous exhalation, you'll also supply fresh oxygen to the region.

Vision and constipation: Hardening of the lens of the eyes (glaucoma) is hastened by the absorption of poisons that originate in the large bowel as a result of intestinal toxemia. Toxemia is a direct result of constipation, and the eyes are quickly affected.

When troubled with anxiety, nervousness, headaches, inability to concentrate—analyze. Chances are, you're constipated. Are you listless, irritable, lacking in energy? Look to your colon. Poisons allowed to accumulate there quickly spread, via the bloodstream, to every part of the body. The answer is not a laxative. The answer is natural grain foods, bran, raw salads—natural laxatives. These foods are the only way to dissolve and remove hardened deposits of toxic wastes lining the walls of the colon! Walk to stimulate glandular function, which stimulates colon activities.

Caffeine: Do avoid all coffee, colas, teas, and other beverages with caffeine, which definitely damages the eyes. Beer and tobacco also should be avoided. Herb teas are excellent, especially eyebright for the eyes.

Sugar and hamburgers: These are two of our most popular food items, but they are dangerous to our health, especially the eyes. Both tend to block utilization of chromium and calcium, so vital for proper vision. Chromium is needed to regulate fluid pressure inside the eye. Calcium prevents muscle tension and spasms. Sugar leaches chromium from the body, while too much protein—hamburgers, steaks, chicken, fish —reduces the body's reserve of B vitamins. This is especially true of hamburgers loaded with animal fats and preservatives.

PREVENTION THROUGH PROPER DIET

Many holistic eye doctors now declare poor nutrition to be a principal cause of eye disease. With the development of the electronic microscope, molecular cell analysis, and microphysiology, doctors can now study blood vessels in the eyes and determine how poor nutrition affects eyesight. They can detect that cells of the retina require more nutrition than any other cells in the body. Thus, the eyes are the first to display symptoms of a poor diet.

A poor diet—too much sugar, starch, and fat—results in hypoglycemia, which means the retina is being denied the fuel it requires for normal functioning. Next, the poor diet brings on arteriosclerosis (hardening of the arteries), which means the arteries in the eyes are affected first. And then there is diabetes. Everyone knows diabetes is linked not only to bad nutrition but also to sight impairment, even blindness.

It is difficult to understand why medical science remains blind to the relationship between nutrition and eyesight when the disease of diabetes clearly indicates what can happen when the diet is deficient. Blindness, diabetes, and diet are clearly interrelated. And millions of cases of impaired vision can be traced to allergic reactions, conjunctivitis, and respiratory infection—all caused by or related to diets high in sugar, flesh foods, and processed starch and low in vitamins and minerals.

Eyesight and Vitamins/Minerals

Time was, not so long ago, when practically the whole world believed all that was required for good eyesight was to take vitamin A—or drink carrot juice, a principal source of that vitamin.

Now we know a bit more. We know you can't isolate one vitamin and expect the best results. It must be united with other nutrients to be fully effective. The eye, a magnificent, complex organ, has a variety of nutritional needs.

The eye is a ball filled with a jelly-like fluid. The tissue surrounding this fluid is called the *sclera*—the whites of the eyes. The front portion of this remarkable ball is called the cornea, which is a transparent tissue.

Light enters through the cornea, passes through the crystalline lens directly behind the cornea, and focuses on light-sensitive cells lining the retina on the back wall of the eyeball. In healthy eyes, operating as nature intended, the cornea and lens bend the light rays as they enter and focus them on the retina, which activates the optic nerve. The optic nerve is the carrier of messages to the sight center in the back of the head.

Some of the light-sensitive cells of the retina are sensitive to color, while others simply detect various shadings of inflowing light. These latter cells, called rods, contain a pigment called rhodopsin, or *visual purple*, which is chemically similar to vitamin A. We have mentioned this previously. Light striking the rods chemically breaks down the rhodopsin, and it can be restored only if a generous supply of vitamin A is present. Without such a supply, the rods cease to function.

The first sign or symptom of the breakdown of visual purple is the loss of night vision. The eye no longer distinguishes colors. Such a deficiency calls for vitamin A. The cornea is also damaged when this vitamin is lacking, but the greatest damage is to the retina. *However*, for vitamin A to be fully effective, vitamin E, a natural antioxidant, must also be present. Vitamin A needs vitamin E for proper absorption in the retina. It also requires zinc, an important mineral. Zinc deficiency can create a faulty metabolism of vitamin A, especially in the retina. Night vision may quickly be restored by the intake of zinc with vitamins A and E.

The very function of sight causes vitamin A to be absorbed and "used up"; just looking at things diminishes the supply of vitamin A, as a car burns fuel. It should be replaced daily. It is the retina that requires a rich supply. It needs and absorbs vitamin A like a sponge. Remember: visual puple, so necessary for night seeing, is found in the retina.

The eye requires good muscle tone, and good muscle tone depends on vitamin C. Vitamin C aids in producing collagen, a gluelike substance that binds cells together. Deficiency in vitamin C could cause blood vessels in the eye to hemorrhage. At least 100 milligrams a day are necessary. Emergency measure require from 250 milligrams up to several thousand daily. More than once, cataracts have completely disappeared simply by adding grapefruit to the daily diet. And vitamin P, or bioflavonoid, seems essential. Deficiency in *potassium* contributes to hardening of the soft eye tissues.

The only way old age can be a factor in failing eye health is that one has had years and years of unwise habits: years of processed food, pasteurized dairy products, white flour, salt, and white sugar products; years of lack of exercise and relaxation techniques. If one eats natural, unprocessed foods, takes proper vitamins/minerals, exercises the eyes, and practices relaxation techniques, the eyes will be as "young" at eighty as they were at eight. Old age itself has nothing to do with vision. Old age itself is not toxic. Eyes, as organs, are ageless.

White sugar and white sugar products are poison, especially for the eyes. People who crave sugar are "-holics," just as much as alcoholics. When you eat too much candy, for instance, you are on a "binge," just as "alcoholic" as the drinker. Sugar leaches vitamin C from the eye tissues.

Riboflavin (vitamin B²) is essential for eye health. It is positively essential for cellular regeneration and for general health, not only for the eyes but for preventing skin diseases and the loss of hair. It seems particularly important in eye health. Dimness of vision, blurring, photophobia, lack of fluidic flow, night blindness, and numerous other disabilities have all responded to riboflavin added to the diet. Cataracts have been known to disappear. Ocular lesions, characterized by bulbar conjunctivitis, lacrimation, burning of the eyes, and failing vision, also have been cured. Usually treatment with riboflavin was coupled with vitamin A therapy. Vitamin A alone did not help, but when coupled with riboflavin, cures were noted, for vitamin A requires riboflavin to be properly absorbed. Rich sources of riboflavin are dried beans, seeds, brewer's yeast, wheat germ, nuts.

Research has clearly established a relationship between cataracts and a low-calcium diet. Vitamin D is essential for proper calcium metabolization, and the best possible source is a moderate exposure to sunlight—not necessarily the sun but sunlight. Since the body is almost totally clad in clothing most of the time, and since smog and pollution frequently block out pure sunlight, it may be a good idea to add vitamin D from a natural vitamin source to your diet.

Live Food and Healthy Eyes

A salad should include from five to eight of the following raw foods, listed in alphabetical order: beets, broccoli, cabbage, carrot, cauliflower, celery, cucumber, endive, escarole, garlic, jicama, kale, lettuce, mushrooms, onion, parsley, peas, pepper, radish, spinach, sprouts, tomato, turnip, watercress, zuccini. To these should be added seeds—sunflower, sesame, and pumpkin—and a shake of kelp powder. A daily portion of sunflower seeds supplies the needed vitamin A. It also acts as an aid to eye infections and inflammation. Before adding any dressing, pour over the salad a small portion of the purest imported olive oil, which coats the vegetable and helps retain their nutrients.

It also has been established that cataracts develop through a calcium buildup. This seeming contradiction is explained by the fact that the body cannot properly metabolize *calcium in unnatural form.* Calcium obtained in pasteurized milk and other processed dairy foods is not a natural calcium. Calcium in its natural form is found in uncooked, untreated foods, unpasteurized milk, or unprocessed dairy foods.

It would appear that to prevent cataracts and other major eye problems the diet must include calcium, zinc, and vitamins A, B², C, D, E, and P. But these should be taken in natural, not synthetic form. A diet rich in natural food will supply many of these essentials, but since most foods have been so adultereated, it seems wise to locate a reliable natural tablet to be taken daily—one made with vegetable or herb sources, not animal. Such a product is difficult but not impossible to find.

Brewer's yeast is an excellent source of vitamin B², which has already been mentioned as being beneficial to the eyes. Brewer's yeast contains a generous supply of riboflavin—which naturopaths have been prescribing as a preventative measure for years! Brewer's yeast is also very good because it contains *all* the B vitamins plus other nutrients. It isn't wise to take isolated vitamin B products. You should always take a supplement containing the entire B family. Cures for several eye problems have been corrected by taking twelve yeast tablets a day.

Gerovital

No book on health and maintaining the energy of youth would be complete without a mention of Gerovital. And if it aids in maintaining the health and vigor of youth, it must also be an aid in maintaining good eyesight.

When I wrote about Gerovital, popularly known as GH3, in a previous book, *The Book of Beginning Again*, the vitamin-drug was illegal in America except in the state of Nevada, because the F.D.A. refused to recognize it as a vitamin and insisted it was a drug. In 1983 it became legal in California.

How did that come about, after so many years of seeking approval of this miracle product? Well, it's had an interesting history: Back in 1951, a doctor in Bucharest, Romania, made medical history. Dr. Anna Aslan, seeking to alleviate the pain of an elderly patient suffering from an injured knee, decided to experiment with injected procaine, plus several other ingredients. So remarkable was his response, she decided to experiment further by using the same formula on all of her aging patients. Not only were their pains slowly eliminated, but they began to display evidence of returning well-being, vigor, and unexplained energy.

Her formula included procaine hydrochloride, a combination of PABA (para-aminobenzoic acid, a B complex vitamin) and DEAE (diethylaminoethanal, a building block of choline, another factor in the B complex). The formula was stabilized with benzoic acid and potassium metabisulfite.

PABA and DEAE work on the glands, hair, and intestines. They also stimulate brain cells against senility and act as antidepressants, both active against stress symptoms.

As her aging patients began to lose symptoms of old age, news of her treatment spread. Her several clinics were filled with clients from all over the world, seeking relief from various illnesses and simultaneously finding symptoms of aging disappearing.

Legalization of GH3 in California came about through the efforts of a group of medical scientists working at the University of California at Los Angeles (UCLA) who performed years of testing, proving that once procaine entered the body, it ceased to be a drug and became PABA and DEAE, two very important and potent compounds of the vitamin B complex (benzoic acid and choline). It finally met the approval of California legislation as a vitamin, not a drug. PABA stimulates beneficent intestinal flora to utilize folic acid and vitamins B1 (thiamine) and K. DEAE participates in manufacturing choline and acetylcholine in the body, both vital anti-aging vitamins. All without the damaging side effects that so often accompany the use of drugs.

GH3 has proved effective for the past thirty years, aiding such afflictions as arthritis, diabetes, ulcers, blood pressure, heart disease, sexual impotence, arteriosclerosis, Parkinson's disease, aging appearance, poor hearing, and in restoring a feeling of buoyant youth—and also in maintaining good eyesight and stimulating new hair growth. It dilates blood vessels, allowing more oxygen to reach the brain.

Perhaps the legalization of this important "youth drug-vitamin" in California means that the barriers restricting its use in this country are beginning to fall. Not being one to enthusiastically endorse a drug, but being aware for years that it converted to anti-aging vitamins in the body, I am most happy that California has made this vital product widely available.

I have used GH3 for years, both as injections and as tablets, and feel I am a living testimonial to its benefits. In my late sixties I feel better than during the years of my youth.

CURES FOR COMMON AILMENTS

Probably the most common eye ailments are nearsightedness, farsightedness, and astigmatism. This section will provide a summary of corrective treatment for these eye disorders, as well as take a look at some other forms of remedies—herbal, natural, folk remedies—and some common misconceptions about the use of drugs to treat eyes.

Corrective Treatment for Vision

Nearsightedness (myopia) is the condition that results when light rays are brought to a focus in front of the retina rather than on the macula lutea, thus producing blurred vision when viewing things at a distance. The treatment is as follows:

1) Blink frequently.

2) Train the eye to focus on one point.

3) Shift.

4) Practice the Long Swing (which is shifting), especially at bedtime.

5) Do central fixation exercises for 5 minutes, then the Long Swing. Repeat the cycle several times.

6) In the myopic eye, the pupil is frequently dilated. These eyes especially respond to sunning. Handball, tennis, Ping-Pong, and badminton are sports to train the myopic eye to use central fixation and shifting.

7) Practice the Elephant Sway.

8) Practice reading a book upside down.

9) Read the letters on an eye-test chart 10 to 20 feet from you without glasses. Read each letter, blinking after each one. Practice at least 5 minutes.

10) Continue faithful daily practice for 1 month; longer for serious cases.

Farsightedness (hyperopia) occurs when rays of light are brought to a focus back of the retina rather than on the macula lutea, thus producing a blurred image in the visual centers. Farsightedness means seeing a distant view easily but finding it difficult to see close objects, such as when reading. Corrective treatment:

1) Blink often.

2) Shift often.

3) Try reading by holding your book about 14 inches away. Focus on one word at a time and blink until it becomes clear. Read for 3 minutes. Rest 1 minute. Just look casually at the whole page, blinking. Increase reading time daily.

4) Practice the Long Swing.

5) Discard your dark glasses except in very special circumstances.

6) Practice reading the letters on an eye-test chart, following the same instructions as given for nearsightedness.

Continue to practice faithfully for 1 month for noted improvement, probably total correction for simple cases. Several months may be required for severe cases.

Astigmatism results when several meridians of the eyeball fail to come together at a single focal point. The lines coming into the eye from a horizontal plane do not meet at the same point as the lines coming from the vertical plane. Ophthalmologists believe this to be a deformity in the development of the eyeball.

But doctors and patients alike have proved the defect to be functional, not structural—a malfunction of muscles, not a malstructured eyeball. The most common muscular defect is caused by unequal tension of the upper and lower recti muscles as opposed to the oblique muscles on either side, causing an abnormal flattening of the eye in one meridian. This could occur only through the malfunction of the extrinsic muscles.

Astigmatism *will* cause headaches, upset stomach, nervousness. These symptoms are far more common than impaired vision. Glasses *do* give relief from the symptoms but certainly offer no hope of correction. The holistic approach is to discover what tremendous stress caused the condition and correct it through relaxation techniques. It occurs frequently during puberty, when the body is undergoing numerous changes. Patient and persistent practice of the Bates system of relaxation—sunning, palming, the Long Swing—has resulted in correction too many times to be denied. But unless one is willing or can give the required time, glasses are the customary answer. Try the following corrective treatment:

1) Blink and shift frequently.

2) Practice the test chart reading according to instructions previously given.

3) Read the chart with one eye covered. Alternate, covering the other eye.

4) As you read the chart, practice the Elephant Sway; blink.

5) Practice Elephant Sway with alternate eyes covered for 5 minutes.

6) Practice reading without glasses. Don't hurry. Blink and read one word at a time. Continue for 10 minutes, holding the book 14 inches from the eyes.

7) Practice just looking at microscopic print, 7 inches from the eyes. Blink often. Look for 3 minutes. Rest 1 minute by practicing the Elephant Sway. Look at print for 3 more minutes. Sway again.

8) Practice the Long Swing faithfully.

9) Sunning is necessary, followed regularly by palming.

10) Play games such as tennis or badminton, or practice with a friend just tossing a ball, for needed shifting and central fixation.

11) Try reading a book upside down.

Herbs and Other Remedies

Certain herbs have long been known to be beneficial to the eyes:

Succus Cineraria Maritima: *Succus* (meaning juice) *cineraria maritima* is a homeopathic remedy (herb) that usually may be purchased at any homeopathic house. Since it is an herb, an herbal establishment may also supply it. It is famous as a preventative or cure for cataracts. It increases circulation in the intraocular tissues—which means more food to the cells and more toxic wastes removed. Instill two drops in each eye morning and night or one drop in each eye four or five times a day. But to be totally effective, blood circulation must be coupled with proper nutrition. And the other channels of the body, such as the kidneys, must eliminate body toxins efficiently.

Eyebright: The very name of this herb indicates its usage and reputation. In recent years it has become even more famous as a means of curing cataracts through an equally famous doctor of naturopathy, John R. Christopher. He created his own "eyebright formula," using the herbs eyebright, goldenseal root, bayberry bark, and red raspberry leaves to which he added cayenne pepper. He marketed this formula as an herbal remedy for eye ailments. As a remedy for cataracts, he suggested:

> 1 or 2 Christopher Eyebright capsules (approximately 1 teaspoon) and 1 cup (8 ounces) distilled water.

Empty the contents of the capsules, or 1 teaspoon, into an 8-ounce teacup. Pour boiling distilled water over it and cover with a saucer. Let it steep from 15 minutes to overnight. Strain, preferably through a piece of white cotton cloth (or wool). When cool, fill a glass eyecup and bathe one eye, blinking and exercising the eye. Discard and fill another eyecup for the other eye.

The eyebath will smart because of the cayenne pepper. Hold the eyecup over each eye to the count of 20, or even longer if cataracts are present. Use one batch of tea for 2 days only; then make a fresh mixture. In the beginning, only 1 capsule to a teacup may be tolerated, working up to 2, and bathing for as long as 5 to 10 minutes for each eye. The tea should also be drunk for quicker results.

One can purchase eyebright herbal capsules at any health food store, but the Christopher formula is completely different. Be *sure* to purchase Dr. John R. Christopher's Herbal Eyebright Formula, also available at health stores. It has been proved to be an excellent means of causing cataracts to be reabsorbed—or cured.

Linseed oil: Before surgery for cataracts became so common, old-time naturopathic doctors used raw linseed oil, purchased at a drug or health food store, as a cure for cataracts or to improve eyesight. The remedy was to drop one drop of linseed oil in each eye every night before retiring. Linseed oil is an excellent source of unsaturated fatty acid.

ALOE VERA AND THE EYES

During my deep muscle massages, my masseur made me aware of an aloe vera product that turned out to be good for the eyes. So I must share my discoveries. This natural aloe vera product is called Aloe Vera Activator and is put out by Forever Living Products. Its principal purposes were as a liquid mixer with the facial mask, as an astringent, or to be applied to insect bites or skin abrasions. But it had found a secondary and far more important use—eyedrops!

It seems that someone had decided to drop the activator solution into her inflamed eyes. Why? Simply because it happens to be pure stabilized aloe vera gel. She was not surprised when it healed her eyes. Others took up the practice, and now the Aloe Vera Activator is widely used as remarkable eyedrops. Perhaps you can buy Forever Living Products from a distributor in your neighborhood—check your local health food store, and refer to the appendix in this book for sources.

I now use the Aloe Vera Activator as eyedrops daily and can add my testimony to that of others. Although I've not yet thrown away my reading glasses, I have found it to prevent burning and itching eyes.

FOLK REMEDIES

In recent years there has been a sudden return to "old home remedies"—folk medicine. Discouraged by emphasis on drugs prescribed by the usual doctor, many have begun to resort to "folk remedies," seeking methods of self-healing. A few are listed below:

A drop of a mixture of eucalyptus, honey, and castor oil in the eye helps to keep the eyes healthy.

Equal parts of fresh lemon juice, distilled water, and pure raw honey. Two drops in each eye twice a day. According to Dr. Som, this remedy cures cataracts.

(The above two remedies should not be cold. I believe, too, their use should be supplemented with good vitamin/mineral tablets to make sure the diet includes calcium, riboflavin, and vitamins B^6, C, and A.)

Aloe vera gel applied to eyes with a dropper. (Be sure to use a glass dropper, not plastic.) Good as a daily eyewash.

Aloe vera gel mixed with wild raw, unrefined honey, applied to the eyes with a dropper 3 times a week at bedtime. Has been known to cure cataracts.

Black eyes—forget the beefsteak theory. Instead apply cold compresses immediately, about 15 minutes every hour.

Purifying the eyes: Insert your little fingers in your ears. Open your mouth wide and close it again. Repeat several times. This opens many channels throughout the head that may be clogged with debris.

Homeopathic cell salt called silicea. For cataracts, 12X potency is suggested. Calc. Fluor (Calcium fluoride) is reportedly excellent. These cell salt minerals can be purchased at a homeopathic pharmacy or a health store.

Brewer's yeast tablets. Four tablets three times a day have been known to cure cataracts.

NATURAL REMEDIES

Oculotrophin: Dr. Som used to prescribe a homeopathic remedy called oculotrophin, which is made from the eyeballs of sheep, pigs and cattle. It comes in tablet form, and you should take one with each meal for three months. The remedy is available through herbalists, naturopaths, homeopaths and holistic doctors, or a homeopathic pharmacy. Oculotrophin has the effect of reawakening or renewing the programming of the eye.

Foot bath: Dr. Som says it may seem strange, but when eye difficulties develop, the problem may be corrected with treatments of the feet. Try soaking them first in warm water containing Epsom salts for 3 minutes, then plunge them into cold water for 1 minute. Alternate back and forth, ending with the cold plunge. Also massage the feet thoroughly. There is a direct connection between the feet and the optic nerve. Pressure on nerves in the feet will stimulate the optic nerve in the brain. This is the secret of reflexology. The water treatment has a similar effect.

Honey treatment: I read an article concerning glaucoma and honey in *Let's Live Magazine* which I've never forgotten. The writer, an elderly man, suffered from glaucoma to such a great degree that he had to wear double, colored glasses. He couldn't read or watch TV anymore. He said he read an article in *Let's Live* by a man who had regained his eyesight after being blind with cataracts for four years. The man had used pure, unadulterated, unheated wild honey in his eyes. The glaucoma victim decided to try this same program. He dropped the honey in his eyes every second night. Six months later, he could read for fifteen minutes and watch TV for an hour. He discarded the colored glasses. Eventually the honey totally removed all inflammation. The sting of the honey drops subsides after a moment.

Vitamin B^2 (riboflavin): In most cases of bloodshot eyes, vitamin B^2 (riboflavin) is indicated. Experts suggest taking 200 milligrams a day for a month; then reduce to 50 milligrams. Vitamin B^6 is also advisable, to reduce muscle tension; and 2,000 milligrams of Vitamin C for 3 days only. Redness could indicate an infection. The above should heal it. If not, see a doctor.

First-aid wash: Here's a good herbal solution to use as a daily eyewash:

    1 tablespoon fennel seed, crushed
    1 tablespoon comfrey root, crushed
    10 ounces of water

Bring the water and herbs to a boil in a small steel or enamel pan. Immediately turn off the heat, cover the pan, and let the mixture steep until cool. Strain through close-woven cheesecloth into a sterile jar. Refrigerate. Bathe eyes with a glass eyecup from one to three times daily. Discard, drink, or pour the remainder over your plants on the third day and make a fresh batch.

Tea bag treatment: Steal away for a moment to relax. On your eyes, place a moist bag of camomile, fennel, parsley, or eyebright tea. It will cleanse and remove shadows.

Filtered seawater: From a sterile dropper bottle, drop 2 or 3 drops of filtered seawater in your eyes night and morning as a daily eyewash. (Purchase from a health food store.) This natural eyewash contains salt, as do our tears, and is a marvelous saline solution for eyes. It also can be taken internally for general health. Epsom salts water is also a good eyewash.

Aspirin: Surprise! Yale Medical School reports that taking from 3 to 4 aspirin daily will delay cataract growth for up to 10 years and in many cases will eliminate the need for surgery.

But aspirin has a bad reputation for stomach disturbances for some people. Four a day could be uncomfortable. Aspirin (2 a day) also has been known to control or prevent heart attack. You may not relish a daily dose of 4 tablets, but you should not hesitate to take 2 if you have a heart condition. Certainly take them occasionally for pain relief, such as headache or arthritis.

Itching eyes: When eyelids are swollen or itch and burn, or when the eyes are watery, there is an indication of a lack of vitamin B^2 (riboflavin). Yeast tablets are an excellent source of all B vitamins.

Circulation: When first waking, squeeze your eyes tightly as you inhale deeply. Hold. As you exhale, blink lightly and quickly. Repeat three times. Then stretch toward the ceiling, hold, and relax. Also take capsicum herb capsules. Capsicum (cayenne pepper) is renowned for improving circulation all over the body. Taken at bedtime, it stimulates blood circulation to warm cold feet and improve sleep, as well as causing a free-flowing bloodstream all during night hours.

Sun reading: Try reading outdoors without your glasses to strengthen eyes. This will bathe your eyes in light rays.

The water cure: Dr. Som believed in the water cure for just about everything, including eye ailments. Get two pans of water, one containing very hot water, the other, cold water with ice cubes. Drop a washcloth into each pan. First apply the cloth from the hot water to the eyes. Hold for 2 or 3 minutes. Immediately alternate to the cloth from the ice water. Hold over eyes for only 1 minute. Repeat the entire procedure three times, ending with the cold pack. The applications prevent congestion. The hot water draws blood to the eyes; the cold drives it away, carrying congestion with it.

The breath cure: Fresh air contains fresh oxygen, and your eyes crave oxygen. Open a window or step outside, perhaps during a TV commercial, and take a deep breath. Then drop forward from the waist, exhaling. Hang loose. Let your arms dangle. Bounce up and down from the waist, head toward the ground. Stand erect, inhale, and repeat three times. Your eyes have had an excellent oxygen bath. Many toxins will be gone. Also your spine will be flexed.

Pinkeye: Conjunctivitis, known as pinkeye, is caused by an irritation of the eye related to bacteria or virus. It causes excessive tearing that, drying on the lashes, especially during sleep, can be very uncomfortable. The eyes are red and swollen and seem to be filled with gritty sand. There also may be a burning sensation. Linings of the eyelids are inflamed. Similar problems can be the result of allergies, creating severe itching. Irritation from chemicals—such as chlorine in swimming pools, exposure to smoke (even cigarette smoke) or smog—can cause similar symptoms.

Use the warm-cold water splashes often. Also place warm wet compresses over your eyes to prevent the fluids from drying on the lashes, and use cold compresses to reduce any swelling. If moisture dries on the lashes, a cotton-tip applicator moistened with water is helpful. Relax with a moist teabag of eyebright tea covering your eyes. Soak a cloth with aloe vera gel and place it over your eyes. If natural methods do not improve the problem within 3 days, see a doctor.

Simple at-home test: If you suddenly find yourself with inflamed eyes, there is a simple test that may prevent an unnecessary trip to the eye doctor. If you have harmless pinkeye, no trip is necessary. But if you have *iritis*, you must certainly see your doctor as soon as possible. Here's how to tell the difference.

Secure a penlight or flashlight. Cover your inflamed eye with your hand. Shine the light directly into the good eye for 3 seconds. If you do *not* feel any pain, you probably have pinkeye, a simple irritation that can easily be treated by salt water solutions and hot-cold splashes of water on your eyes, or with the natural methods described above. If you *do* feel pain in your covered eye, you probably have iritis and should see your doctor at once.

Pinkeye is a harmless inflammation of part of the eyeball and inner eyelid, whereas iritis is a serious inflammation of the iris, the colored part of the eye. In the home test, when light is directed into the good eye, the pupils of both eyes contract. If iritis is present, pain results. If no pain results, it is a fair indication that the iris is not involved.

Headache and eyes: "You have headaches? You probably need glasses!" How often have you heard this? We have all been brainwashed to connect headache with the need for glasses, totally ignoring the millions of aspirin taken for headache daily by those who already wear glasses.

It's true that when a headache strikes, we don't see as well. But cause of the temporary loss of vision may be a poisoned colon, which can certainly impair the eyesight. Don't put on glasses to prevent headaches without first cleaning out the colon, the usual culprit. A "bad" colon results in "bad" eyes, which can never be made "good" with glasses. Of course, you can see better. But your eyes will still stay "bad" until the colon is again "good."

How sad it is to see children fitted with glasses, without a thought to the probable diet of sugar, candy, ice cream, cokes, hamburgers, greasy potato chips, hot dogs, cold cuts, processed milk. To put glasses on children is to doom them for all the years ahead. Glasses *never* permanently correct headaches. Eyestrain may be accompanied by a headache, true, but is never the sole cause of a headache.

What is common, however, is the headache caused by ill-fitting lenses. Glasses commonly cause headaches, not the other way around. If you have headaches, tired eyes, and eyestrain, check your reading habits. Does a bright light reflect in your eyes, or do you have the light coming properly over your shoulder? Do you prop up on one arm to read? Do you hang your head forward over your book?

Do practice the Long Swing prior to bedtime to insure a relaxed eyeball all during the night. If your eyes *are* causing eyestrain and headaches, this will usually correct the problem. It can also cure insomnia.

Treatment for simple eyestrain: Try the following:

1) Bathe your eyes in hot, then cold, water.

2) Blink frequently.

3) Shift frequently.

4) Practice the Long Swing faithfully, especially just before bedtime.

5) When driving a car, do try blinking, shifting, and seeing with central fixation.

Healing an inflamed or infected eye: First administer drops of castor oil directly into your eye. Next soak a tea bag—preferably eyebright, but almost any mild tea would do—in castor oil and place it over your eye as a poultice. Lie down and cover the eye and poultice with an ice bag. The eye should be healed in a few hours. If not, see a doctor.

Chemical burns: When any chemical contacts your eyes, flood them with water continuously for at least 15 minutes. Hold your head under the faucet, stand in a shower, or pour water into your eye. Be sure your eyes are held wide open. Do not use an eyecup or bandage your eyes. See your doctor.

Cuts and punctures: Bandage your eyes lightly. Do not wash with water or apply pressure. Do not attempt to remove an object stuck in your eye. See a doctor immediately.

Fasting according to Dr. Som: Fasting is often needed to give the digestive apparatus a complete rest, but Dr. Som did not approve of long fasts. Nor did he think it advisable to fast on water alone for a long period of time. He suggested fasting one day on liquids such as pure water, fruit juices, and vegetable juices—a glass of one every 2 hours—then eating light solids the second day, such as fruit or a small green salad. Drink liquids between meals. Or you may wish to stay on liquids for 2 days and solids the third day for a period of 2 weeks.

This will attain a purification without the danger, hungers, or frustrations of a rigid fast. Two days on liquids and one day on solids for a week or so is an excellent method of fasting. With this method, enemas are not necessary. Food taken on alternate days keeps the bowels in good condition, requiring neither artificial stimulation nor mechanical action.

To Dr. Som, it was imperative to drink alkaline vegetable juices. He much preferred them to fruit juices, which can make the system too acidic. But if fruit juices are to be used, they should be alternated with alkaline vegetable juices. Such a fast should go far to clean away many eye problems.

Natural eyewash: Dr. Som recommended a homemade eyewash. Here is his recipe: Hold 1 tablespoon of table salt in an open flame and brown it. Mix it with 2 tablespoons of Epsom salts. Dissolve the mixture in 7 ounces of distilled water. Apply to the eyes with an eyedropper. For a plain salt water eyewash, mix 1 teaspoon of sea salt in 1 cup of distilled water. Bathe the eyes with this mixture or drop it into them with a glass dropper. If too strong, reduce salt to ½ teaspoon.

Massaging the eyes: After bathing your eyes, close them and place your first, second, and third fingers over the eyeballs and massage them gently. Then vibrate your eyes with your fingers by making rapid tapping movements over them, stimulating them gently.

Seeds and carrots: Of course Dr. Som also recommended eating sunflower seeds, caraway seeds, taking vitamin A, and drinking carrot juice.

Apple poultice: I have also known Dr. Som to apply a poultice of decomposed apple to the eyes. He simply scraped or peeled an apple and let it decompose in the air until it turned brown. Then he placed the brown decomposed apple over each eye.

HEALING WITH LIGHT

Normal health depends on the energy of light. Light contains life force. Confine humans to total darkness and the life force begins to ebb away. White light is the most powerful of all light energies. Future medicine points to the time when doctors will prescribe certain wavelengths of light instead of drugs and chemicals.

The eyes are our greatest organs of light. A great intake of light is necessary for the complicated mechanical processes in the brain on which all our senses depend—especially sight.

As we have already discussed, the eyeball resembles a small rubber ball 1 inch in size, except that it is filled with a transparent jelly-like substance instead of rubber or air. A clear watery fluid floats near the front part. Unlike the round rubber ball, a section bulges out on the surface of the front part. It is called the cornea. It resembles transparent glass. Acting as a lens, it collects light rays.

The iris is the part that contains the color essence. The black pupil is a hole in the center of the iris. It is the action of the pupil, a complicated system of very small muscles, that determines the amount of light allowed to enter the eyes. It opens or shrinks, without conscious thought, to control the inflow of light. In bright sunlight the pupils contract to little more than the size of a pinhead, obstructing the inflow of too much light. In a dark area they dilate to allow more light to enter, instinctively responding to the need for light in order to see. Light, reflected from everything around us, is of many different wavelengths, producing various colors.

The nerve endings of the retina (the inner lining of the eye) are separated by what is called pigmentation. This pigment automatically changes its form according to the degree of light or darkness to which we're exposed. The basic pigment, as already explained, is known as *rhodopsin,* or *visual purple.* It is the presence of rhodopsin that enables us to see in comparative darkness. The electricity of light bleaches rhodopsin—which then becomes *fuscin*—enabling us to see in daylight. So in daylight, we depend on fuscin pigments, and in darkness we depend on rhodopsin.

Our awareness of the necessity to make a rapid switch becomes obvious when, for instance, we go immediately from a well-lighted lobby into a darkened theater. It requires a few moments for the fuscin to transmute to rhodopsin. When we exit from the dark theater, we are momentarily blinded until the rhodopsin again becomes fuscin.

It is important to maintain the quality of the basic rhodopsin pigmentation of the retina since its quality is also reflected in our daylight pigmentation, fuscin. One practice to assure its quality is to make sure our bedrooms are dark during our sleep hours. Darkness during sleep assures restfulness for the eyes. Even a small degree of light can penetrate the thin covering of the eyelid, often creating tension during sleep and disturbing total relaxation so needed for visual perfection.

Walking in the evening under a dark night sky would be beneficial for training eyes to see better in darkness, as would time spent looking outward through the window of an unlighted room or sitting quietly in a totally dark room. This allows the basic rhodopsin pigmentation of the retina to recharge after exposure to a whole day of bright sunshine or artificial light. Too much light is tiring. Palming is excellent to maintain pigmentation balance, especially in restoring the visual purple necessary for night-seeing.

Visible Light Ray Therapy

Visible ray, or color, therapy has proved beyond question that separated wavelengths of light energy are a natural remedy for many eye problems. Reflection of color and light is often very beneficial to the eyes, especially in the case of cataracts, glaucoma, muscle paralysis of the eyeball or other muscles around the eyes and the retina, even correction of nearsightedness, farsightedness, and astigmatism.

When we refer to red, orange, yellow, green, indigo, blue, and violet rays, we are actually referring to different wavebands and wavelengths of indirect electricity. These light rays operate on low, average, or high voltages just as electric motors do. All types of electric motors must be fed with predetermined voltages of electricity. The "electromechanical" activity of the eyes—and the processes of vision in the brain—require similar voltages.

Nearsighted people are invariably amazed at how well they can see without their glasses in outdoor bright sunlight. And often, after only one treatment with stimulating color rays, the patient is amazed at how much easier it is to read a distant test chart. When cataracts are diagnosed, color ray therapy should be begun immediately. The orthodox method is, or has been, to allow the cataract to grow until it "ripens" for surgical operations, which usually means a long waiting period of gradually worsening eyesight. All patients, but especially those who are otherwise normally healthy, inquire why their eyes have become so affected. There are constitutional disorders, and often mechanical causes, such as having resorted to reading glasses too early in life.

The Treatment

Red and orange rays are stimulating, yellow only mildly so; green is sedative, while blue and violet are depressive. The longer the wavelength, the warmer the ray. The shorter the wavelength, the cooler the ray.

Secure pieces of colored glass—yellow, purple, violet, red, green, orange, and blue. Begin with the yellow glass and look at the sun through it for 20 to 30 seconds, blinking steadily. Then close your eyes for about a minute and repeat with the other colors. Do this once or twice every day early in the morning and late in the afternoon. If you own a slide projector, insert a colored glass slide and allow the colored ray to focus fully on you for 5 to 10 minutes. Select the colors indicated for your particular need at the moment.

For cataracts and hardening conditions of the eyeball, use purple glass. If the eyes are inflamed, use blue glass. Remember to close and relax your eyes between each treatment. Use red glass to stimulate circulation in the eyes and green to sharpen the vision.

One of the greatest authorities on visible ray color theraphy is R. Brooks Simpkins of England. He writes of his incredible success in restoring eyesight in his book *Visible Ray Therapy of the Eyes.*[3] He started his experiments using only a flashlight containing two 2.4-volt flashlight batteries. The

[3] R. Brooks Simpkins, *Visible Ray Therapy of the Eyes*, (Rustington, England: Health Science Press, 1963).

light of the flashlight was placed behind the transparent colored sheet, 6 inches from the eye.

Later he built a machine called a *Fixoscope*, which contains a 12-volt, 12-watt projector into which the patient gazes at a certain color. Mr. Simpkins uses red for 10 minutes, green for 10 minutes, and then 5 minutes of blue. Red is used for stimulation; green disperses congestion of wastes; and blue relaxes and relieves tension. Serious cases are treated 5 days a week for 25 minutes. Two days of rest are important. He reports incredible success with cataracts and glaucoma and in less severe cases of farsightedness, nearsightedness, and astigmatism. In other words, he has helped people discard their glasses. It may be possible to purchase a Fixoscope from him for your home use. A letter of inquiry might reach him at the address provided in the appendix.

Following is a list of documented improvement through ray therapy:

1) purification of aqueous fluids in the eye;

2) improvement of circulation;

3) sedation of the nervous system;

4) increase of harmonic flow;

5) utilization of calcium and phosphorus by the body;

6) normalization of blood sugar;

7) reduction of blood pressure;

8) stimulation of the thyroid gland;

9) stimulation of antibodies, causing the body to resist infection;

10) increase of leucocytes, thus strengthening the capacity to overcome bacterial infection;

11) stimulation of heat in deeper tissue structures by the deeply penetrating longer wavelengths, thus eliminating congestion;

12) release of lymphatic stagnation, resulting in dilation of blood vessels in circulation and the supply of blood;

13) increase in retinal pigmentation (when retinal pigmentation is deficient, the eyes become unduly sensitive to bright light);

14) improvement in off-focus eyes or crossed eyes.

Visible ray, or color, therapy is a natural remedy, and its astonishing benefits await the exploration of all ophthalmic practitioners. We are only now beginning to understand the mystery of light—especially in medicine. Such knowledge has become essential to the preservation of our eyes and the visual processes in the brain. Those seeking such knowledge almost immediately realize that the total visual mechanism is of an electronic nature.

DRUGS AND VISION

Unnatural drug therapy is unnatural for the body—therefore, in most cases, harmful to the eyes. One of the most damaging drugs is *cortisone,* a steriod. It is linked without question to the development of cataracts.

Any kind of steroid therapy is to be avoided. You should especially avoid *prednisone,* a steroid hormone, used for rheumatic disorders, asthma, blood disorders, certain cancers, inflammatory problems. It is usually administered over a period of time. *Quietidin,* a tranquilizer, has been linked to the development of cataracts.

Pregnant women should totally avoid the use of drugs and injections, even those used in immunization for measles, chickenpox, smallpox, diphtheria, or whooping cough, since these drugs may affect the developing eye structures. In most cases, the use of these drugs is irreversible.

Sugar, while it is not widely recognized as a drug, has a most destructive affect on the entire body. It is especially destructive to vitamin assimilation, thus being indirectly responsible for many diseases. While sugar itself probably cannot be held responsible for the development of cataracts, nevertheless, the fact that it is detrimental to many other bodily functions points strongly to its adverse affect on the eyes. What is detrimental to the body must also be detrimental to the eyes, since the eyes are an important part of the bodily functions.

Sodium nitrate is a definite culprit, and its use should be studiously avoided. It occasionally appears in certain wines, especially those from Italy. It is almost universally used in red meats to maintain the color and to prevent spoilage. Bacon, cured meats, hot dogs, luncheon meats, corned beef, and all meats not absolutely fresh are laced with sodium nitrate and nitrite. People who eat these foods habitually are constantly exposed to sodium nitrate and its dangers, not only to the eyes but to the entire body.

Smog! The population of the entire world is familiar with the fact that exposure to heavy smog and air pollution contributes to burning and eye discomfort. While there is no proof that these atmospheric conditions contribute to cataracts, there is obvious evidence that they do affect comfort and result in burning and inflammatory conditions.

Laxatives containing liquid paraffin are to be avoided, including mineral oil.

● ● ●

On the positive side, it must be said that the drug industry occasionally does come up with a drug product that helps mankind. Such is the new drug *Timolol*, used to aid glaucoma patients. Timolol, which has been tested by several teams of researchers, seems not to have side effects—not even pain, headaches, or allergies.

Timolol has so far had only beneficial effects—preventing blindness in the majority. Before Timolol, other drug medications blurred the vision, caused the development of cataracts or kidney stones, or caused painful discomfort, such as innumerable allergies. Timolol, now in drops, seems the answer to the prayers of those who, unaware of a diet-exercise natural life-style, become victims of glaucoma, the most unfortunate of all eye diseases.

Another drug of popular use in glaucoma is *Diamox*. It rapidly eliminates fluid from the eye as well as from the entire body. Removal of fluid also decreases tension and arrests the damage being done by inner pressure. Inquire concerning any side effects.

CHELATION THERAPY AND NEW AGE MEDICINE

I first heard of chelation therapy during one of my hideaway treks to the desert to write another book. Always alert to new breakthroughs in holisitc medicine, I began asking questions. My inquiries led me to the office of Dr. Robert Harmon, renowned throughout the Palm Springs area as a holistic physician and sought by patients nationwide as an expert in chelation therapy. He consented to an interview so that I might share with my readers much of his expertise. The following interview between myself and Dr. Harmon will be of great interest to all those interested in health, not only for the eyes but for the whole person:

Earlyne: I've heard so much about chelation therapy, all of it good. But I'd like to hear from a medical doctor just how it works.

Dr. Harmon: Well, the first thing we notice is that it rapidly dissolves calcified calcium deposits that have adhered to the walls of the arteries. It is this hardened chalky substance that creates "hardening of the arteries," or arteriosclerosis. As these deposits begin to break up and move out of the body, a chain reaction begins. The parathyroid glands begin to be reactivated. These are two small glands located in the throat near the thyroid. As one grows older, our modern life-style invariably causes these glands to slow down, and this is a major cause of aging. During the chelation treatments, the parathyroids become active again and, through them, all other glands are stimulated.

Earlyne: The overweight problem that usually besets those in middle and later years—could it be caused by a sluggish thyroid?

Dr. Harmon: Yes indeed, and we always give our chelation patients a thyroid extract because we want the metabolic rate to be increased.

Earlyne: Does one lose weight during chelation treatments?

Dr.Harmon: Invariably! Patients always lose weight.

Earlyne: Do you also place them on a diet?

Dr. Harmon: Oh yes! But we don't restrict the amount of food, only certain items—no salt, no sugar, no processed dairy products, and so on.

Earlyne: How about the vegetarian?

Dr. Harmon: The treatments will be doubly effective for the vegetarian.

Earlyne: Let's talk about youth and the parathyroids again.

Dr. Harmon: Well, the parathyroids become active again— and if there is any one gland that can bring about rejuvenation, it's the parathyroid. Even members of the medical profession don't realize this. As we age, we lose calcium out of our bones and our teeth. It accumulates metastatically—or erroneously—in the soft tissues, the muscles, the joint tissues, the walls of the arteries.

Earlyne: We lose it because of inactive parathyroids?

Dr. Harmon: Exactly. Now calcium in our body, like everything else in the universe, must flow. When it becomes static, then there is a leaching process. It leaches collagen out of the bones. It seeks another place to rest; usually it's the soft muscle tissue. Then we say we're aging. Now when you reverse this and begin a calcium flow back into the bones and the teeth, back into the cells, then we have a form of rejuvenation. It's a simple nontoxic process. Actually, we are injecting into the bloodstream an amino acid. It is called ethylenediaminotetraacidic acid (EDTA), and it is a substance of very low toxicity—approximately one-fifth that of aspirin. We encourage people to take a minimum of twenty therapies because with less than that we are not always able to produce the results we want. In a few cases, such as in removing metallic poisoning—lead, mercury, cadmium—we have had patients who required sixty or more treatments before all these toxic metallic substances were removed from the intercellular fluids.

Earlyne: Do you have some way to discover if it is all out of the system?

Dr. Harmon: Oh, easily. We take a bit of hair or nails for analysis; the hair is easiest to obtain in sufficient quantity. And with a new technique, the "argon-plasm process," we can determine exactly the levels of twenty-eight different minerals or metals in the body.

Earlyne: In other words, what you're saying is that in addition to "rejuvenation" and reversing the hardening of the arteries, we are also removing from the body the toxic metals that have accumulated through pollution and other undesirable aspects of modern life.

Dr. Harmon: Toxic metals, yes; we all have them to some extent.

Earlyne: That seems tremendously important to me.

Dr. Harmon: I believe that's why people sometimes, after only three or four treatments, say, "Doctor, I feel so much better; I haven't felt this good in many years." Now we haven't had time to "rejuvenate" the arteries at that point, but we have removed quite a load of metals, and these people are beginning to feel a resurgence of vitality. They feel as if they are coming back to life.

Earlyne: How about the iron, Doctor? We need iron. Does it take the iron out?

Dr. Harmon: The iron is ninety-five percent locked into our red blood cells, and it cannot be touched by the EDTA, not in the slightest. Just the undesirables are removed from the bloodstream.

Earlyne: What is actually happening, Doctor? One hears so many things. The popular notion is that blood is being drawn out of the body, cleaned, and then reinserted. Surely this isn't correct. You've already mentioned the process, but could you elaborate?

Dr. Harmon: Yes, of course. What we are doing is inserting a solution into the bloodstream, a solution of mineral salts that are naturally contained in your body, plus the amino acid (EDTA) I mentioned. It is a very well known substance, as a matter of fact; small amounts are contained in at least twelve hundred foods, so you know it's nontoxic. This amino acid has the property of grasping calcium and heavy toxic metals and bringing them right out through the kidneys, the intestines. This grasping is called chelation.

Earlyne: What was the other thing you put in?

Dr. Harmon: Mineral salts—cell salts that are natural to the body. We also put in vitamin C; that speeds up the process. We put in several other things: trace minerals that we want to replenish and some important vitamins. We also put in a bit of procaine. This is popularly known as Gerovital or GH3.

Earlyne: Well, we put all these good things into the bloodstream, but what is happening to the body now?

Dr. Harmon: The amino acid solution flows into the bloodstream and then out through the kidneys and intestines, bringing with it all the toxins, the dissolved chalky deposits we wish to bring out of the body through the chelating process. It is a beautiful process and one that we have been employing successfully for many years. As a matter of fact, it has been in use since 1935. In all the tens of thousands of cases that we have treated, we have not had one serious side effect or undesirable reaction to this therapy. That must make it unique; I don't know of any other modality about which we could make that statement. I believe that chelation therapy comes closest to the most sacred part of the Hippocratic oath; that is, "Do ye always good, but at least do no harm." If all physicians nowadays would practice under this great oath, what a wonderful thing that would be for the patients and the doctors and everyone else in the health care delivery system.

Earlyne: How often are the treatments given?

Dr. Harmon: Well, twice a week is the schedule we prefer. If the patient has a time factor, then it can be given three times a week safely. If you have to make a trip or for some other reason miss a treatment or two, it doesn't set you back; the process goes right on.

Earlyne: Doctor, tell me about the treatment. What will I experience? Where will the solution be administered?

Dr. Harmon: It is fed into the bloodstream by inserting a tiny needle—almost like a hair—into either arm, in any vein that can be reached so that you are comfortable. You recline in a big chair, the feet elevated, the arm resting quietly on a pillow. You sleep, read a book, visit with a neighbor, or just relax for three hours. It isn't painful, only a slight needle prick.

Earlyne: If someone such as I sought chelation—and I have no major health problems—would the treatments act as a preventive measure?

Dr. Harmon: Certainly—and that, after all, is the very best kind. Chelation enables the blood to circulate as it did in your youth. So while chelation does not make one *look* young again, it certainly can make one *feel* younger again because the arteries are as they were in younger years.

Earlyne: Your literature mentions that chelation effects the macula and the fovea centralis. Have you ever known anyone to discard glasses?

Dr. Harmon: Oh yes! As a matter of fact, I myself did! I used to wear glasses day and night for reading and for all vision. I haven't worn them for years now.

Earlyne: Do you attribute this to chelation therapy?

Dr. Harmon: In part.

Earlyne: Marvelous! Did you just find your eyesight getting stronger and stronger?

Dr. Harmon: What I found was that my glasses were getting far too strong. They hurt my eyes to wear them. So I decided that instead of getting weaker glasses, I'd just discard them altogether. This I did—and my eyes immediately began to strengthen. Now I have unbelievably good vision.

Earlyne: How old are you now?

Dr. Harmon: I'm fifty-six—soon will be fifty-seven. I wore glasses from the time I was in first grade. I had a lot of trouble because they used to call me "Four Eyes." I was the only kid in school who wore glasses. Now I haven't worn glasses in at least seven years.

Earlyne: You give chelation therapy only partial credit, Doctor. What else contributed to your restored eyesight?

Dr. Harmon: The rays of the sun.

Earlyne: Oh, I have an entire section on sunning in my book. I'm delighted to have you endorse it.

Dr. Harmon: I'm a living example of sunning for the eyes. Let me describe my method. One must look directly at the sun for at least one or two minutes just as it comes over the horizon in the morning. Right at it, blinking repeatedly.

Earlyne: But so many advise against looking directly at the sun.

Dr. Harmon: I'm saying, yes, look directly at the sun, blinking, for two minutes in the early morning. I have done it with very good results. My mother is ninety. She has been sunning like this for years and wears glasses very little, if at all. Her eye doctor keeps warning her she'll get cataracts if she continues such practices, but she doesn't. Some of her friends have—those who don't do sunning—but not her.

Earlyne: Can you explain something about the ultraviolet rays?

Dr. Harmon: Well, Earlyne, let me say that I believe the eye—in fact, the whole human organism—was designed to operate and function in a daily contact with full-spectrum light from our sun. That development, of course, took millions of years, and during those millions of years the creatures that eventually evolved into homo sapiens functioned in full-spectrum sunlight.

Nowadays we spend our day reading tiny ciphers on white paper—even far into the night by artificial light—and I believe fluorescent lighting may be the most unnatural and harmful of all, unless you purchase the full-spectrum tubes made by Vita Lite.

Sunlight, when measured by the spectral photometer, forms graphically what we may call a bell-shaped curve of infrared to ultraviolet. At the very top is the color green at approximately fifty-five hundred Angstrom. You'll notice how many things in our environment are green and how most people respond favorably to this color. Around twenty-seven to thirty-one Angstrom we have a long-wave ultraviolet. This is an extremely important part of the spectrum, not only to the eye but to the entire body, because of its stimulation of the pineal gland, which is directly connected to the retina and passes messages through to the pituitary, both through hormone production and directly through nervelike fibers. It is this very long-wave ultraviolet band that is completely filtered out by most glass and plastic substances, and remember that most of us spend our lives behind one, two, three, or four sheets of glass or plastic when you count windows, eyeglasses, contact lenses, et cetera.

Earlyne: Earlier you mentioned eyedrops. Can we discuss these more?

Dr. Harmon: We use specially formulated eyedrops of a diluted sterile saline solution to which enzyme substances are added. The patients drop it into their eyes twice a day. We are seeing fantastic results—even with cataracts and glaucoma.

Earlyne: Could one use the drops just as a health measure, even if one has no particular eye problem?

Dr. Harmon: I would not recommend them for prevention in the absence of a definite treatable problem. But for prevention, I can tell you that eyebright is a marvelous herb, used as an eyewash or taken internally. Another suggestion of extreme importance is vitamin D—calciferol. I give my eye patients this important supplement.

• • •

My interview with Dr. Harmon left me with some very valuable information on eye treatment. At the end of the interview, Dr. Harmon said he would be more than happy to forward literature and information to interested readers. His address has been provided in the appendix.

I was so impressed with chelation therapy that I decided to embark on the program of twenty treatments, three times a week. My only health problem at the time was a muscle spasm on the left side of my neck that caused painful disturbance from time to time. But throughout my life I have sought programs of rejuvenation and methods for retaining youth. In many of my writings and seminars I have shared my findings with my readers and listeners.

Since I was involved in writing this book at the time I discovered chelation, I thought it a good idea, even though I was enjoying good health, to experience the therapy personally, the better to report on it.

My first reaction was a headache on the day following the first treatment, caused by the stirring up of many toxins flowing out of the body. But following the headache, I experienced a remarkable elevation of energy—too obvious not to be noticed. This pattern—the treatment, the headache, the energy uplift—repeated itself following each of the first few therapies. The neck muscle spasm improved.

But during the three-hour sessions I heard many of the other patients sharing stories of their improvements. Most were people who had experienced drastic health measures, such as severe heart attacks, even bypass surgery. Some had severe kidney problems and swollen legs; some had eyes almost blind with macular degeneration—oh, too many ailments to mention.

In each case, each patient gloried in relating his or her improved condition. Gone were the chest pains. Thrown away were the nitroglycerin tablets. I could not help but be amazed. I realized I could not measure the benefits of chelation by my own personal history, since I was enjoying fairly excellent health. True judgment could be made only as I "eavesdropped" on the conversations all around me. It sounded like a study in miracles, as each patient, without the least solicitation, extolled the wonders of his or her improvement. I never heard one single negative report.

But throughout these comments I heard repeated mention of the therapist there who gave deep muscle massage. Those enjoying the greatest and most dramatic improvement seemed to be those who coupled their chelation with massage. And, too, I had heard Dr. Harmon frequently recommend it as an adjunct for more rapid recovery.

Because I still suffered some discomfort with the neck muscle spasm, I decided to try it. That's when the rapid improvement really began. Gone were the headaches, gone was the spasm pain. The headaches did not return as my treatments progressed. I found myself feeling incredibly well, with unbelievable energy. I found that the neck spasm returned if I neglected the deep muscle massage, but with only slight discomfort. By the time I completed the twenty chelation treatments, coupled with massage, I can truthfully say I felt better than when I was young. I can certainly recommend it and hope it would be sought as a preventive measure, rather than following tragic health loss, especially heart problems and surgery.

IF YOU MUST WEAR GLASSES . . .

Being realistic, I realize millions of people wear glasses; but being a woman, plus a teacher, I feel duty bound to help my readers look as beautiful or handsome as possible while wearing glasses. So let's discuss color and styles. The right color of your eyeglass frames depends on your hair color.

Black hair: black frames or other dark colors. Or silver. Avoid crystal (clear) and light colors.

Dark brown hair: medium-brown frames, gold or twotone with the top line darker. Avoid black, dark gray, silver.

Medium brown: light tortoise, light brown, gold. Avoid black, dark gray, dark brown, silver.

Blonde: gold, light brown, light tortoise, beige, crystal. Avoid all darker shades.

Gray: medium or light gray frames, silver, or gold. Avoid black, dark brown.

Take an honest friend with you for selection of eyeglass frames. Try on many shapes and sizes. Wear your usual makeup. Avoid flashy styles.

For a *round face,* choose oval frames. They are longer than they are wide. Avoid round frames. Choose angles.

For a *long face,* choose round frames or angled frames, wider than they are long.

For faces with undereye puffiness, choose round frames. Avoid thin wire frames.

If you *must* have tinted lenses, choose amber with a slight rose shade. But remember, tinted lenses block out healthy and healing sun rays.

Don't wear rimless glasses habitually in the sun. Heat accumulates around the rim, burning the skin on the cheeks under the eyes. Constant irritation of repeated daily wear could cause serious skin diseases, even cancer of the tissues. Discard such glasses immediately, or wear them only in the shade or at night.

Contact Lenses

For those who *must* use glasses, contact lenses are a blessing. They can be purchased in either soft or hard lens material. Many whose professions demand that they not wear eyeglasses—such as the athlete, the actor/actress, the sportsman, the lecturer—find contact lenses indispensable. Others wear them simply because they are a definite improvement over glasses.

Contact lenses have now been perfected to the point of being wearable up to three weeks without the need to remove them—and then only to be thoroughly cleaned. This abolishes the daily in-out procedure. This special lens is made to float loosely enough to allow the flow of natural fluids to keep the eye moist. Those who can wear them are indeed fortunate, but they should still practice an eye improvement program.

Those who wear contact lenses should take a generous supply of vitamin B6. The eye needs to be moist in order to wear contacts successfully. Some eyes become deficient in natural moistrue from tears and tear ducts due to a lack of vitamin B6. With such dryness, contact lenses become uncomfortable. Vitamin B6 corrects the problem. It also prevents muscle cramps and spasms, not only in the eye muscles but in the leg muscles, which cramp when B6 is needed. Take from 50 to 200 milligrams a day. Some require 500 milligrams.

To find a lost contact lens, stretch a piece of nylon stocking over the end of a vacuum cleaner hose. The suction will recover the lens. It will be clearly visible on the stocking.

Why Not Reading Glasses?

A book written by a leading ophthalmologist suggested that if one had no serious eye difficulty, he or she should buy dime store reading glasses for reading. He said they were as good as those prescribed by an expensive doctor. I checked this with my own eye doctor. He agreed. It seems they correct defective vision, allowing you to read clearly. They will not damage your vision and you'll save a lot of money.

Take a newspaper or magazine to a store with you, and keep trying on reading glasses until you find a pair comfortable for you. They will cost about ten dollars. A trip to an ophthalmologist, optometrist, or optician's office could cost up to $150. In their offices, they speak mysteriously about grinding lenses to fit your prescription, but no grinding whatever is done there.

There are three major optical suppliers that grind all the lenses for everyone. They also grind the lenses sold in the inexpensive dime store reading glasses. There is no exact prescription in these reading glasses, so if you find a lens that's a quarter of an optical unit greater or less than your prescription, no damage is done. The same is probably happening with your expensive glasses.

All the optometrist or optician does is examine your eyes and write out a prescription. Then he orders the lenses from one of the three major suppliers, who looks through his stock, selects lenses as close to your prescription as possible, and ships them to your optician. When the lenses arrive, they are fitted into the frames of your choice. The lenses may fit your prescription no better than those bought in a dime store. So as long as your only need is reading glasses—magnifying glasses—why not try the dime store kind? Your eyes will not be harmed.

BREAKTHROUGHS IN
MEDICAL TECHNIQUES

Eye has not seen nor ear yet heard of the marvels science has waiting for a humanity that needs them. If you have tried all the techniques in this book, or if you started on this kind of therapy when the condition of your eyes was already too far advanced, then the following medical breakthroughs may be of some benefit to you. The advances now being made by medical science will be welcomed by those who either rely on such approaches, or by those who need this kind of care.

As I said at the beginning of this book: Do what you can. *Don't be stubborn.* If you come to the realization that you cannot help yourself, please see your doctor. Eyesight is one of our most precious gifts. Many people become stubborn about homeopathy and new age techniques—but don't let yourself go blind because you didn't take care of a pressing condition. Speak to your eye doctor about the following possibilities, as one of these therapies may be just what you need.

Lens Implant

One of the most important developments in eye-science in the past ten years is the use of *intraocular* implant lenses for cataract sufferers. This process involves removing the clouded crystalline lens from behind the pupil and inserting or implanting in its place a plastic prosthetic lens.

This procedure restores vision to the patient without the need for thick uncomfortable glasses—which tend to magnify things all out of proportion—or contact lenses, which, even though more comfortable, are often tedious to insert daily. With the intraocular lens implant, none of the problems of spatial disorientation or abnormal peripheral vision associated with cataract glasses occur. This surgical procedure, a major operation, requires the technological expertise of a skilled surgeon and seems to be very effective in removing cataracts and restoring lost vision in one operation.

With intraocular lenses, it is now no longer necessary for patients to wait for cataracts to mature. Nor is it necessary to wait for the growth of a cataract in one eye to "catch up" with a more advanced cataract in the other eye. Once a cataract develops in one eye enough to become a problem, the lenses in both eyes may be removed and the new plastic lenses implanted, so that vision in both eyes may be equalized and restored. A cautious physician, however, usually operates on the faulty eye first, waits to determine developments, then proceeds with the other eye.

A method called the *"emulsification and aspiration"* technique is now widely used to remove cataracts. It involves removing the crystalline lens by liquefying it and removing the liquefied lens through an aspirator.

The conventional method of cutting out the lens consists of making a 180 degree incision around the cornea to expose the lens. It is then removed by touching it with a *cryogenic* (super cold) probe, to which the lens adheres. With the newer method, a much tinier incision is required in the cornea. The cataractic lens is removed by means of a tiny hollow needle, the tip of which vibrates 40,000 times a second against the lens. The vibration causes the lens to liquefy. This liquid is then drawn off, or aspirated, after which the new plastic lens is implanted. The healing time required is much less than with the older conventional method of cataract removal as much less radical cutting is involved.

Radial Keratotomy

Radial Keratotomy (or RK) is a new technique now being developed that eliminates or reduces myopia (nearsightedness) and astigmatism. In this amazing procedure, the ophthalmic surgeon creates between four to sixteen micro-fine incisions radically on the periphery of the cornea. These minute incisions, which extend partway through the cornea, are outside the optical zone of vision, so they do not affect or interfere with sight. But the incisions—together with the normal fluid pressure of the eye—create enough pressure on the cornea to cause it to flatten. The flattened cornea focuses images clearly on the retina in the back of the eye, enabling the patient to enjoy restored vision without glasses or contact lenses.

This incredibly simple procedure was first developed in Russia, moved into Brazil, then into the United States. It is an out-patient procedure that requires less than a half hour to perform. This procedure is still in the experimental stages, and requires precision laser instruments. You will probably find that it is not yet available to you—nor is it advisable to proceed with such an operation while it is still so new. Look to 1988 to show some advancements in this technique.

Epikeratophakia

Epikeratophakia is a procedure available to those who are farsighted. As with many medical terms, this one is borrowed from the Latin. *Epi* means "on top of," *kerato* refers to the cornea or clear outer surface of the eye, and *phakia* means "lens." So this mouthful of a word means "a lens on top of the cornea"—or a lens constructed of reshaped corneal tissue.

The farsighted patient has developed a cornea that is cone-shaped, resulting in blurred vision. The usual corrective measure up to now has been to prescribe glasses, contact lenses, or a nonreversible corneal transplant. Epikeratophakia offers an alternative.

In this procedure, a donor cornea is reshaped to fit over the patient's own cornea. Once placed, this reshaped corneal tissue can optically correct the faulty vision of the patient's own cornea. Or better still, the patient's own faulty cornea is removed, reshaped and refitted into the eye.

Again—I stress caution. This is another procedure in the experimental stages, and you'll find that you'll be hearing more about it as its success rate continues.

Expertise Required

While lens implants are now a fairly common procedure, RK and Epikeratophakia are still new. If possible, wait until they have been further developed. You should know about these procedures, but you should also be aware of how new they are and therefore risky—it seems to me that many of us fall victim to doctors who prescribe surgical procedures because they are itching to "try them out." Always seek the finest ophthalmic surgeon in your area—and get another opinion. All three of these procedures are out-patient processes, requiring from fifteen minutes to an hour and a half. But they do need the attention of an expert ophthalmologist.

Oculinum

A cure for cross-eyes and off-focus or "wandering eye," without surgery. Oculinum is a new and widely hailed drug for treatment. When a patient has crossed eyes, the muscles that control eye movements are imbalanced so the eyes can be looking in different directions. The brain blocks out the images coming from one eye, so the patient may slowly lose vision in that eye.

A tiny portion of Oculinum is injected in the stronger eye muscle, which temporarily paralyzes it, causing the muscle on the opposite side of the eye to work harder at focusing and balancing. The procedure is painless and can be done in a doctor's office.

A Cure for Dry Eyes

An amazing new capsule cures "dry eyes," an affliction often found in arthritics. This is an inability to produce tears, so important in natural cleansing, purifying, and moistening the eye. It occurs mostly in women. The common symptoms are itching, burning, and redness. If untreated, the patient could experience severe drying of the cornea—which again could lead to infection and corneal ulcers.

The new treatment consists of inserting a tiny capsule or sliver of gel into the lower eyelid that lubricates thoroughly.

Before this gel discovery, patients often found it necessary to use eyedrops constantly—whereas the new gel needs insertion only once a day. Since 90% of such patients are women, could this affliction of "dry eyes" be caused by some frequently used eye cosmetic—such as old contaminated mascara, eyeshadow or liner pencils? Just a thought....

Cyclosporin A

This is a safe treatment for *uveitis,* an inflammation of the interior of the eye, which results in visual impairment. This new drug stimulates the body's own immune systems. Previous drugs produced serious side effects, such as diabetes, high blood pressure, ulcers, and loss of hair. (It might be better to suffer with uveitis!?) This new drug is supposed to produce only "minor" side effects. Do inquire what these "minor" side effects are. You may prefer Dr. Christopher's herbal eye wash—which has none, and usually cures such afflictions.

A Cure for Lost Eyelid Control

There is a new treatment for those who have lost control of the eyelids—suddenly they clamp shut uncontrollably. The lids shut so tightly that even vigorous pulling cannot open them.

The new procedure is to open a small incision in the cheek (under anesthesia) over the area where the facial nerve begins to branch. A tiny battery-operated nerve stimulator helps find the exact defective nerve branch, which is then cut and removed, producing "total relaxation of the muscles yet allowing normal blinking to operate."

This "new procedure" requires much further investigation, it seems to me. It certainly does not eliminate the *cause* of such an affliction. Proceed cautiously. Why not simply try palming first? The culprit cause *could* be emotional tension.

Nyctalux

A pill called *Nyctalux* is available in France to aid night vision. Taken half an hour before a trip begins, the drug reduces the blinding effect of dazzling oncoming headlights. It also enables a driver to see objects in the dark more clearly. Nyctalux accelerates the ability of the light-sensitive pigment in the eye to return to normal after having been impaired by bright lights. The great advantage of the pill is that the drug has no side effect. In France it is considered a medical breakthrough. Your American doctor may be able to obtain it or a similar medication. Or, again, try palming, which restores night vision.

Ultrasound and Fluorescein Photography

Other late developments in eye care include the use of *ultrasound* to detect and remove foreign objects from the eye. And the use of *fluorescein photography*—a method of photographing the retina—to diagnose cancer and other conditions.

Ultrasound makes it possible to locate non-magnetic as well as magnetic objects. The ultrasound instruments are also equipped with miniature forceps to remove the object. New camera equipment together with fluorescent dye now make diagnosis of serious conditions more certain. The dye is injected in the arm. The retina is photographed as the dye passes through the tiny blood vessels of the eye. If a malignancy is present, many blood vessels will be apparent. But other conditions will not. Thus differentiation is possible.

Testing for Strokes

There is now a simple test that can determine whether or not you are a potential stroke victim. It is performed in the office of an ophthalmologist and requires no more than five minutes.

The patient lies on a table. A tonometer—an instrument for measuring the pressure of glaucoma—is placed gently on the eyelid, to which a surface anesthetic has been applied to prevent any discomfort. With the tonometer resting on the eyeball, the physician presses on the carotid artery located on the side of the neck. This stops the flow of blood to the eyeball for a few seconds and causes the pressure inside the eyeball to decrease.

If it drops at a normal rate and rises at a normal rate, this means the blood supply to that side of the brain is normal. But if, after applying pressure to the carotid gland, no change is detected in the pressure of fluid in the eyeball, there is a clear implication that a blocked artery is preventing blood from reaching that side of the brain. The same test is applied to the opposite side of the head.

If a test proves a possible blockage, do change your diet and take every step to dissolve the blood clot that could cause a stroke. The test is called *carotid compression tonography*.

Laser Treatment for *SMD*

A common eye disease for many people over fifty is called *senile macular degeneration* (SMD). It affects the macula, the yellowish dot in the center of the retina that is crucial to such activities as reading, sewing, driving. A miraculous new laser beam treatment is saving the eyesight of many so afflicted. The laser treatment seals off abnormal bleeding that affects the macula and leads to severely impaired vision.

The macula lutea, as we've already explained, is a small, yellow pigmented spot located directly behind the pupil. In the center of this spot is found the important fovea centralis. The fovea is the area of greatest visual acuity of the eye. Bates drills and swings are designed to keep the fovea free from tension—which should also correct problems with the macula.

Try the following daily test to check for signs of SMD. Pick out a door frame, a telephone pole, or anything with a rigid straight line. Cover one eye and see if the line is still straight. Repeat with other eye. If the line appears bent or distorted, or if a blank spot appears, see a doctor immediately. The laser treatment for SMD is relatively comfortable for the patient, is usually done in a doctor's office, and costs about $1,000 for each eye.

Aid for Diabetics

A safe and effective laser treatment has recently become available to diabetics and promises to reduce the risk of blindness. Called *laser photocoagulation*, it uses laser light to destroy excess blood vessels that build up in the eyes of diabetics. It is usually completed within a thirty minute session. Some patients require a return session. The cost ranges between $1,000 and $2,000.

• • •

Discussing new procedures with my ophthalmologist, I was surprised to hear him declare that by 1992 glasses would be obsolete. Well, perhaps. But there are many who fear surgery enough to still insist on glasses.

However, being the eternal optimist, I hope you will seek to avoid all these medical approaches and opt for perfect vision through diet, exercise, and thoughts of love, service and prayer. Establishing the best possible pattern for well-being will manifest perfect eye sight. Only then can the eyes truly reflect the imprisoned splendor—the soul.

APPENDIX

Products, Suppliers, and Sources

Through the years, I have accumulated a wealth of information on natural products that seem to be beneficial to the eyes, as well as people to contact for supplies and services. I share that information with you here. The first place you should always check for products and remedies is your local health store or homeopathic pharmacy. Company addresses frequently change, and your local distributor should know where to point you for more information on how to get the products mentioned in this book.

Aloe-Vera Activator, and other Forever Living Products: write to Sonya and Wilbur Brown, 43540 Texas Street, Palm Desert, CA 92260.

Chelation therapy: Write to Dr. Robert Harmon, Desert Holistic Health Center, 43576 Washington Street, Palm Desert, CA 92260.

Color therapy: There are several color therapy experts. There are many healers who are working with color therapy. Three that I can recommend from personal experience: R. Brooks Simpkins, 644 Kenton Road, Middlesex, England (you can also write to him regarding information on the Fixoscope); Rev. William L. Asher, Jr., PO Box 955, Black Mountain, NC 28711; and James V. Goure, United Research, PO Box 1146, Black Mountain, NC 28711.

Fanie: An excellent line of beauty products. Of principal interest is the eye cream. It not only diminishes and prevents wrinkles around the eyes but, since it contains niacin, also acts as a blood activator to improve circulation around the eyes. Available through Dr. Valjean McGinty, Oma Enterprises, 255 North El Ciel Drive, Suite 369, Palm Springs, CA 92262.

Homeopathic remedies: Write to Standard Homeopathic Pharmacy, PO Box 61067, Los Angeles, CA 90061; or Borneman Homeopathic, 1208 Amosland Road, Norwood, PA 19074.

Herbalife products: offers a vitamin-mineral tablet made completely of herbs among their products. Primary distributor is Dr. Valjean McGinty, Oma Enterprises, 255 North El Ciel Drive, Suite 369, Palm Springs, CA 92262.

Schiff's products: offers a whole line of health care products. They particularly offer a one-a-day vitamin/mineral tablet that I especially like. It's free of wheat, yeast, corn, sugar, and starch. It has a base of rice and soy. Schiff's is available at most local health stores.

Vege-Homo products: for vitamins, minerals, and other nutritional supplements. Available through most health stores.

Wachter's organic sea products: Write directly to Wachter Products, 360 Shaw Road, South San Franscisco, CA 94080. A note of inquiry will bring literature and a price list to you.

INDEX